The United Nations was not created to take mankind to heaven, but to save humanity from hell.

Dag Hammarskjöld

United Nations Secretary-General 1953–1961

"TO SAVE HUMANITY"

What Matters Most for a Healthy Future

Edited by

Julio Frenk and Steven J. Hoffman

OXFORD
UNIVERSITY PRESS

OXFORD
UNIVERSITY PRESS

Oxford University Press is a department of the University of Oxford. It furthers the University's objective of excellence in research, scholarship, and education by publishing worldwide.

Oxford New York
Auckland Cape Town Dar es Salaam Hong Kong Karachi
Kuala Lumpur Madrid Melbourne Mexico City Nairobi
New Delhi Shanghai Taipei Toronto

With offices in
Argentina Austria Brazil Chile Czech Republic France Greece
Guatemala Hungary Italy Japan Poland Portugal Singapore
South Korea Switzerland Thailand Turkey Ukraine Vietnam

Published in the United States of America by
Oxford University Press
198 Madison Avenue, New York, NY 10016

Library of Congress Cataloging-in-Publication Data
To save humanity: what matters most for a healthy future / edited by Julio Frenk and Steven J. Hoffman.
p. ; cm.
ISBN 978–0–19–022154–6 (hardback : alk. paper)
I. Frenk, Julio, editor. II. Hoffman, Steven (Steven J.), editor.
[DNLM: 1. World Health—trends. 2. Climate Change. 3. Delivery of Health Care—trends. 4. Health Policy. 5. Internationality. WA 530.1]
RA441
362.1—dc23
2014043556

1 3 5 7 9 8 6 4 2
Printed in the United States of America
on acid-free paper

CONTENTS

CONTRIBUTORS

Fazle Hasan Abed
Founder and Chair, BRAC

Rebecca Affolder
Special Adviser, Office of the UN Special Envoy on Ebola

Irene A. Agyepong
Lecturer, University of Ghana

Recep Akdag
Former Minister of Health, Republic of Turkey

Sudhir Anand
Professor, University of Oxford

Michelle Bachelet
President, Republic of Chile

Joyce Banda
Former President, Republic of Malawi

Julia Belluz
Health Reporter, Vox.com

Seth Berkley
CEO, Gavi, the Vaccine Alliance

Ela Bhatt
Founder, Self Employed Women's Association, India

Agnes Binagwaho
Minister of Health, Republic of Rwanda

Michael Bloomberg
Founder, Bloomberg Philanthropies

Albina du Boisrouvray
Founder, FXB Foundation and FXB International

Irina Bokova
Director-General, UNESCO

Larry Brilliant
Senior Advisor, Skoll Global Threats Fund

Gro Harlem Brundtland
Deputy Chair, The Elders

Felipe Calderón
Former President, Mexico

Ray Chambers
Special Envoy for Financing the Health MDGs and Malaria, United Nations

Gerald L. Chan
Co-Founder, Morningside Group

Margaret Chan
Director-General, World Health Organization

Helen Clark
Administrator, United Nations Development Programme

Bill Clinton
Former President, United States of America

Paul Collier
Professor, University of Oxford

Francis S. Collins
Director, US National Institutes of Health

Nigel Crisp
Member, UK House of Lords

Suraya Dalil
Former Minister of Public Health, Islamic Republic of Afghanistan

Sally C. Davies
Chief Medical Officer, UK Government

Esther Duflo
Professor, Massachusetts Institute of Technology

Mark Dybul
Executive Director, Global Fund to Fight AIDS, Tuberculosis, and Malaria

Carissa F. Etienne
Director, Pan American Health Organization

Paul Farmer
Co-founder, Partners In Health

Richard Feachem
Director, UCSF Global Health Group

Harvey V. Fineberg
President, Gordon and Betty Moore Foundation

Colleen M. Flood
Professor, University of Ottawa

Julio Frenk
Dean, Harvard T.H. Chan School of Public Health

Thomas R. Frieden
Director, US Centers for Disease Control and Prevention

Laurie Garrett
Senior Fellow for Global Health, Council on Foreign Relations

Melinda Gates
Co-chair, Bill & Melinda Gates Foundation

Amanda Glassman
Senior Fellow, Center for Global Development

Paul Glasziou
Professor, Bond University

Tore Godal
Special Adviser on Global Health, Norwegian Ministry of Foreign Affairs

Lawrence O. Gostin
Professor, Georgetown University

Teguest Guerma
Former Director-General, Amref Health Africa

Angel Gurría
Secretary-General, OECD

Jane Halton
Secretary, Australian Department of Finance

Margaret A. Hamburg
Commissioner, US Food and Drug Administration

Katharine Hayhoe
Associate Professor, Texas Tech University

David L. Heymann
Head, Chatham House Centre on Global Health Security

Steven J. Hoffman
Associate Professor, University of Ottawa

Arianna Huffington
President and Editor-in-Chief, Huffington Post Media Group

John P. A. Ioannidis
Professor, Stanford University

Jay Ireland
President and CEO, GE Africa

Elton John
Founder, Elton John AIDS Foundation

Mustapha Sidiki Kaloko
Commissioner for Social Affairs, African Union

Angélique Kidjo
Founder, Batonga Foundation

Jim Yong Kim
President, World Bank Group

Felicia Knaul
Director, Harvard Global Equity Initiative

Anthony Lake
Executive Director, UNICEF

John N. Lavis
Professor, McMaster University

Alan Lopez
Professor, University of Melbourne

Adetokunbo O. Lucas
Adjunct Professor, Harvard T.H. Chan School of Public Health

Graça Machel
Founder, Graça Machel Trust

Mathura Mahendren
BHSc Candidate, McMaster University

Michael Marmot
Professor, University College London

Malebona Precious Matsoso
Director-General, South African Department of Health

Anne Mills
Provost, London School of Hygiene and Tropical Medicine

Suerie Moon
Lecturer, Harvard T.H. Chan School of Public Health

Chaeli Mycroft
Ability Activist and Co-Founder, The Chaeli Campaign

Sania Nishtar
Founder, Heartfile

Anders Nordström
Ambassador for Global Health, Swedish Ministry for Foreign Affairs

Ngozi Okonjo-Iweala
Minister of Finance, Federal Republic of Nigeria

Gorik Ooms
Researcher, Institute of Tropical Medicine Antwerp

Zulma Ortiz
Health Specialist, UNICEF Argentina

Trygve Ottersen
Postdoctoral Fellow, University of Bergen

Sean Penn
Founder and CEO, J/P Haitian Relief Organization

Navanethem Pillay
Former High Commissioner for Human Rights, United Nations

Peter Piot
Director, London School of Hygiene and Tropical Medicine

Thomas Pogge
Professor, Yale University

Michael E. Porter
Professor, Harvard Business School

Mariana Mota Prado
Associate Professor, University of Toronto

K. Srinath Reddy
President, Public Health Foundation of India

Zain Rizvi
JD Candidate, Yale Law School

Judith Rodin
President, Rockefeller Foundation

John-Arne Røttingen
Director of Infectious Disease Control, Norwegian Institute of Public Health

Simon Rushton
Faculty Research Fellow, University of Sheffield

Richard Sezibera
Secretary-General, East Africa Community

Rajiv Shah
Administrator, US Agency for International Development

Kenji Shibuya
Professor, University of Tokyo

Michel Sidibé
Executive Director, UNAIDS

Akinwande Oluwole "Wole" Soyinka
Laureate, Nobel Prize in Literature

Jonas Gahr Støre
Leader, Norwegian Labour Party

David Stuckler
Professor, University of Oxford

Larry Summers
President Emeritus, Harvard University

Keizo Takemi
Member, Japanese House of Councilors

Christy Turlington Burns
Founder, Every Mother Counts

Kent Walker
General Counsel, Google Inc.

All views and opinions contained in this collection of essays are those of the individual contributors writing in their personal capacities and do not necessarily represent the views or opinions of their respective organizations.

INTRODUCTION

We edited this book to share powerful ideas from some of the world's most thoughtful persons because we believe our shared destiny depends on all of us, everywhere, being engaged and doing our part.

In September 2000 the United Nations convened the single largest gathering of world leaders ever for a Millennium Summit. The objective was to chart the future of international development. Health was high on the global agenda: AIDS was scourging Africa, thousands of women died each year in childbirth, and billions lived in malnourishment and poverty. Solutions were said to exist for each of these global health challenges, but progress was slow because of insufficient political will and financial resources to fully address them.

The outcome of the summit, the Millennium Declaration, was later organized into eight Millennium Development Goals (MDGs): (1) eradicate extreme poverty and hunger; (2) achieve universal primary education; (3) promote gender equality and empower women; (4) reduce child mortality; (5) improve maternal health; (6) combat HIV/AIDS, malaria, and other diseases; (7) ensure environmental sustainability; and (8) forge global partnerships for development. Twenty-one targets and 60 official indicators were then devised as a way of operationalizing the broad goals and tracking progress over time. Each was to be achieved before the end of 2015.

The MDGs were revolutionary in their focus on outcomes rather than process, and how they offered time-bound measurable definitions of success rather than vague aspirations. They have been widely credited with mobilizing unprecedented financing for fighting global poverty and engaging the full range of government, civil society, business, and philanthropic partners. But the MDGs were not crafted without controversy. From a content perspective, the goals created winners and losers, focusing attention on some issues and not others. The goals focused on *average* gains, which could be concentrated among the best-off individuals, instead of *equitable* gains that either target the least well-off or are shared fairly across society. From a process perspective, discussions to set the goals, targets, and indicators did not attract nearly the level of public participation that has characterized the current round of debates on the upcoming post-2015 development goals.

While it is complex to tease out their specific impact, we do know that the 25 years since the MDGs' 1990 baseline has been a time of unprecedented human development. With three of eight MDGs directly focused on health, international development funding in this field increased from $5.82 billion USD in 1990 to $31.3 billion USD in 2013. The numbers on achievement are also astounding. Child mortality has been cut by 47%, maternal mortality by 45%, and the spread of HIV/AIDS, malaria, and other diseases is starting to reverse.

The world's response to global health challenges has been more successful over the past 25 years than during any other similar-length period in human history. Yet future progress is anything but certain. We are currently experiencing one of the most profound health transformations that has ever been seen. Wealthy and poor countries alike face a multitude of new risks now that globalization has eroded any remaining illusion about the protective effect of national borders. Pandemics spread between countries within hours instead of years; improper use of antibiotics anywhere generates microbial resistance everywhere; agriculture has become a single worldwide market with food supply lines globally integrated; environmental degradation and climate change are occurring at increasing speeds. Societies are not all progressing along the epidemiological transition in a linear and irreversible manner, from acute infections to chronic conditions; instead, the 80% of people who live in developing countries face a juxtaposition of old and emerging problems.

Despite best intentions, the existing institutional architecture for global health has proven inadequate for addressing these challenges, especially in the face of a conflicted world that is multidimensionally fractured by income, government capacity, social values, research needs, and industrial interests, to name a few. Interdependence has reached such a level that even the wealthiest countries cannot by themselves control all the factors that affect the health of their populations. Decisions are increasingly being made not only in local communities and national capitals but also in opaque assembly halls in New York and Geneva, and in the private offices of pharmaceutical giants, international organizations, and academic institutions in Beijing, Boston, and London. These decisions affect health but span across many other sectors, including the environment, finance, human rights, migration, security, and trade. Making matters even more complex, the global health system itself is now fragmented across the hundreds (if not thousands) of global health organizations that now exist.

The need for renewed reflection and imaginative thinking on the future of global health is made apparent by the most fundamentally unacceptable reality of our time: that so many people still suffer from diseases, conditions, and risks that we know how to address in a cost-effective way. According to United Nations figures, 2.5 billion people live without basic sanitation, 870 million suffer from chronic undernourishment, and 768 million rely on unsafe drinking water sources. A staggering 222 million women lack access to effective contraception, 52 million mothers each year experience labor without skilled attendants, and 6 million children die annually from avoidable causes. One in every nine girls in developing countries gets married before her 15th birthday. There are 1.2 billion people living in extreme poverty.

The deep inequalities and injustices of our world threaten economic development, global security, and human rights. One must only consider that Americans born today can expect to live 79 years, while Angolans can expect only 51 years of life.

These challenges and disparities—wholly preventable—block efforts to achieve the peaceful and prosperous future that everyone deserves and desires. We realize that this future is not a fixed destination but an unpredictable journey. In the process of building it, we can take inspiration from the words of legendary United Nations Secretary-General Dag Hammarskjöld: "The United Nations was not created to take mankind to heaven, but to save humanity from hell." The unacceptable conditions under which so many human beings are born, live, and die imposes on all of us the obligation to act with what another legendary figure, Dr. Martin Luther King Jr., called the "fierce urgency of now."

The title of this book tries to capture this imperative of redressing avoidable suffering as the foundation for a fair future. Now that the global community is deeply engaged in the search for shared development goals after the 2015 MDG deadline, there has never been a more opportune time to identify what matters most for a healthy future and chart a path for getting there.

* * *

This book features perspectives from nearly 100 persons who are among the most eminent and interesting in the world. About half are leading global health thinkers, while the other half are celebrated luminaries from cognate disciplines, sectors, and fields. About half are leading researchers, some of whom work in the tallest ivory towers, the riskiest level-4 biosafety labs, or the most dangerous humanitarian field settings. The other half are renowned global decision-makers and opinion leaders who rule the corridors of power and shape global reality as we know it, including heads of government, United Nations agencies, multinational companies, media outlets, and global philanthropies. A few contributors are younger, already making their mark and representing some of the best from Generation Next.

Each contributor was invited to prepare a 300- to 800-word essay offering their honest thoughts on the single most powerful idea, the single most important unanswered question, or the single most transformative insight they believe more people need to know in order to improve global health over the next five decades. Contributors were not directed to write on specific topics; each contributor chose his/her own. This means that by reading this book, we get a sneak-peak into the collective consciousness of leading figures and a primer on current world events based on what some of today's top intellectuals, decision-makers, celebrities, and young leaders are thinking. Contributors were asked to write for an educated general public audience with no citations, although we think these essays will also be of great interest to students and specialists in global health, international affairs, public policy, and related fields alike. We also asked contributors to write essays in their personal capacities, reflecting their own opinions and not necessarily representing the views of their respective organizations.

Our selection of contributors was careful and deliberate. The overarching goal was to achieve diversity of leading perspectives across *geography*, *gender*, and *generations*. This wasn't easy. Indeed, the difficulty of the challenge we faced highlighted to us the inequities that persist along these three dimensions. People who are from poorer countries, female, and younger do not yet have the same opportunities that will lead to distinctions like global citizenship awards, science academy fellowships, humanitarian citations, World Economic Forum invitations, United Nations advisory positions, Nobel prizes, or listings among *Forbes* magazine's 72 most powerful people, *Foreign Policy* magazine's top 100 global thinkers, or *Time* magazine's 100 most influential people—all of which served as important pools from which potential contributors were drawn. We hope that changes. But in the meantime, we did our best: out of 96 contributors, 38 are from developing countries, 41 are women, and 11 are under 40 years old.

The diversity of ideas found in this book matches the diversity of its contributors. There are some clear themes. Bill Clinton, Anthony Lake, and Rajiv Shah focus on child health; Carissa Etienne, Paul Farmer, Michael Marmot, and Larry Summers on global health equity. Margaret Chan, Katharine Hayhoe, and Srinath Reddy argue for action on climate change; Fazle Hasan Abed, Joyce Banda, and Angélique Kidjo for gender equality. Michelle Bachelet, Mark Dybul, and Simon Rushton prioritize leadership, while health-care delivery is discussed by Jay Ireland, Jim Yong Kim, and Michael Porter. Tom Frieden, Amanda Glassman, Angel Gurría, and Kent Walker excite us with big data; Francis Collins, Esther Duflo, John Ioannidis, and Alan Lopez with the potential of science. Larry Brilliant and Laurie Garrett write about pandemics; Seth Berkley and Harvey Fineberg about vaccines; and Sally Davies and John-Arne Røttingen about antimicrobial resistance. Larry Gostin, Trygve Ottersen, Navi Pillay, and Michel Sidibé enlighten us with matters of rights and responsibilities. The two of us, and John Lavis, offer strategies for better, evidence-based policymaking.

But for every clear theme there was also a novel dream: Irina Bokova encourages education, Felipe Calderón beckons bigger health budgets, Melinda Gates hones in on human-centered design, Jane Halton talks truth to big tobacco's power, Arianna Huffington supports self-renewal, Ngozi Okonjo-Iweala discusses diet, Elton John calls for compassion, and Chaeli Mycroft demands the realization of disability rights.

And that's just a sampling of 48 essays. This book contains 48 more. We hope you enjoy reading them all and participating in this re-imagination of our shared destiny. With your help, these powerful ideas—and those of your own—can inspire post-2015 global development and a healthier future.

We thank our contributors, editors, colleagues, staff, students, and families for their generosity that made this team effort possible. We owe you debts of gratitude.

Steven J. Hoffman and Julio Frenk

"TO SAVE HUMANITY"

Chapter 1

Harnessing Women's Agency

FAZLE HASAN ABED

Women, when provided with the right opportunities, have the power to solve many of today's intractable problems.

Women's role in health and development is essential, and my colleagues at the Bangladesh Rural Advancement Committee (BRAC) and I have realized their importance time and time again in our work. When we created BRAC in 1972 to support returning refugees in the aftermath of Bangladesh's War of Liberation, we thought our help would only be required for a limited period. We thought the need for relief would be short-lived and that the government would be equipped to take on the more onerous development work to lift people out of poverty, illiteracy, and disease, toward a dignified life. Relief efforts were not sufficient, however, and it quickly became clear that rehabilitation and development were very much a part of the equation. Four decades later, the need for nongovernmental efforts is still relevant and BRAC continues to serve millions of poor and disadvantaged people.

Originally, BRAC chose to work mainly with men, but the limitations of this approach soon became obvious. If BRAC was to change the parameters of development, it had to engage with women at all levels. For example, we had set up several health centers and trained male paramedics locally, but this was short-lived as the doctors were reluctant to work in remote areas; they had greater interest in setting up private practices that would be more lucrative for them. The male paramedics also had limited acceptance of dealing with the specific health needs of women. We then started training local women as community health workers (CHWs), figuring that they were likely to stay in the villages and would be more willing to address the health issues of women and children. We have been very satisfied with their work, and the strategy has now been scaled up to the point that BRAC supports over 95,000 CHWs in Bangladesh, as well as in other countries such as Afghanistan, Sierra Leone, and Uganda. In a study conducted by Swedish investigators, it was demonstrated that there was a 26% reduction in the mortality rate for children under the age of 5 in Ugandan villages where the BRAC model of women CHWs was implemented. By reaching poor and marginalized women and their families, CHWs have helped to solve some of the more intractable problems in health-care delivery.

Tuberculosis, for example, affects people in their most productive age. Yet, even when treatment was available, many people didn't follow the recommended therapy. To address this challenge, BRAC began involving CHWs in identifying tuberculosis patients and providing drugs under their direct supervision, a strategy we used before it was officially recommended by the World Health Organization. BRAC-trained CHWs now administer medicine to over 80 million people in Bangladesh and other countries, achieving cure rates greater than 93%, with less than 1.5% of patients unaccounted for in follow-up.

Similarly, diarrhea from multiple causes has always been a major cause of mortality and morbidity in Bangladeshi children. Since the late 1960s, oral rehydration therapy (ORT) has been shown to be a very effective low-cost treatment for most cases of dehydration from diarrhea. But most villagers in Bangladesh did not know how to prepare and use it. We trained women CHWs to teach mothers how to make and use a home-based ORT of salt, sugar, and water. Teams of women went from village to village teaching ORT to nearly 14 million mothers through an innovative system of education and program management. Thanks to these CHWs, the uptake of ORT in Bangladesh is now the highest in the world, and watery diarrhea is no longer a major killer of our children.

In recent times, the CHWs have further extended their work in dealing with maternal and newborn health problems. They provide antenatal, postnatal, and essential newborn care in rural areas and urban slums and refer maternal and newborn complications to local health facilities or hospitals. In providing instruction on maternal and child nutrition, these workers have been instrumental in improving both maternal and child health.

A recent series of articles about Bangladesh in the medical journal *The Lancet* is a testimony to the remarkable progress the country has achieved over the past few decades, particularly in health. In addition to women's direct involvement in health programs, women have taken on important roles in many other developmental activities, which have either directly or indirectly contributed to the health of the population, especially for women and children. These include some of the world's largest microfinance programs that have helped reduce rural and urban poverty; a community-based education program in which 70% of the students are girls; and income-generating and poverty-reduction programs specifically directed toward women. These programs have also prepared many women to work in the ready-made garment sector that is now a mainstay of the Bangladeshi economy. Women as CHWs, microfinance borrowers, teachers, garment workers, and local entrepreneurs are leading their families and the nation on a path toward better health, social awakening, and development. Women are leading us into the future.

Fazle Hasan Abed is the founder and chairperson of BRAC and is a recipient of the World Entrepreneurship Forum's Entrepreneur for the World award.

Chapter 2

Democratizing International Development

REBECCA AFFOLDER

The democratization of development assistance for health is an important trend that is set to help improve global health in the coming decades.

The international development field is becoming democratized on a scale and depth like never before. There are two main reasons for this mega-trend. The first is the Internet. It has changed the communications landscape and increased information flow. It has broken down traditional barriers to entry in the field of global health and has promoted the emergence of new actors. By enabling like-minded people and organizations all over the world to connect and mobilize, Web-based services like email, Twitter, the blogosphere, Facebook, and other social media have amplified the individual and collective voices of civil society. Individuals now find it easier to participate in local and global dialogue. When an individual becomes aware of the existence of other supporters, this greatly increases his or her confidence and promotes coalition-building. These grassroots campaigns often then find their way into the mainstream media. The BBC's regular "Trending" column reports "buzz" that is being generated on Twitter.

The increased symmetry of information flow has made it more difficult to suppress activism. In the global health arena, this presents an opportunity for previously disempowered members of society to actively push for change. Avaaz, a global citizen movement, tackles corruption and human rights abuses through online activism. This model could be applied to a range of health and human rights issues.

Furthermore, electronic communication enables more efficient collaboration and information-sharing, irrespective of geography. At the end of 2014, the number of Internet users worldwide reached three billion, representing a doubling of African users from 2010. Mobile phone subscriptions soon will reach seven billion. This ensures people can stay informed and demand more from those who purport to act on their behalf.

The Internet has also promoted a growing culture of transparency and an increased demand for the tracking of results and resources. The World Health Organization has led a drive to promote and improve health information systems and accountability. Increasingly, this is generating a culture that fosters innovation and builds commitment to producing data as a global good. Organizations or collaboratitions like Countdown to 2015, Gapminder.org, and the Institute for Health Metrics and Evaluation are generating and sharing quantitative data, which they make freely available through their websites.

The second reason we're seeing democratization in the international development field is the proliferation of new players—nongovernmental organizations (NGOs), philanthropic and corporate foundations, and businesses engaging in emerging markets. NGOs are far more significant in terms of their contribution than they were just 20 years ago, and funding from private philanthropy has increased from $0.5 billion USD in 1990 to $6 billion USD in 2011. With the number of global billionaires now topping over 1,600, this trend is expected to continue. NGOs have also increased their overseas health spending 10-fold during the same period.

New entrepreneurial players are on the field too. Visionary change agendas are inherently risky. Political leaders can find it challenging to drive ambitious change because of the reputational risk of failure and pressure from those who are invested in the status quo.

This provides an opportunity for entrepreneurial players who have a greater appetite to take or underwrite risk. It enables them to seed "big change" concepts by making early-stage catalytic investments. This has parallels with venture capitalism and creative disruption in the business world.

There are many examples of success using this strategy. The Bill & Melinda Gates Foundation leveraged impact by acting as a "lead investor" Gavi, the Vaccine Alliance, thereby galvanizing funding contributions from others. (RED) has raised $250 million in product sales and has mobilized widespread public awareness in the fight against HIV/AIDS.

There is also increased democratization of development funding. The Internet has also enabled micro-payment fundraising. This has not been limited to political fundraising, like the famous example of Barack Obama's US Presidential campaign in 2008. Catapult is the first crowdfunding platform dedicated to the equality of women and girls worldwide. The Po1 (Power of One) campaign enables donation and disbursement tracking for malaria tests and treatment in Zambia.

Opportunities abound for increased entrepreneurial risk-taking and citizen-generated movements in global health. Tobacco-related deaths each year, currently at six million worldwide, are projected to reach eight million by 2030. Savvy marketing campaigns to promote lifestyle changes are expensive and require constant modification. The long fight for sexual and reproductive health and rights will be bolstered through increasing collaboration with grassroots movements. The increased speed at which data can be generated and shared will equip decision-makers to better target scarce resources.

The democratization of international development is important. It will help us ensure that global health keeps improving.

Rebecca Affolder is Special Adviser to the United Nations Secretary-General's Special Envoy on Ebola and former Global Health Adviser in the Executive Office of the United Nations Secretary-General.

Chapter 3

Systems Thinking

IRENE A. AGYEPONG

> We need to do away with the illusion of a compartmentalized world where linear quick-fix solutions work and, instead, encourage thinking that accounts for interconnectedness, complexity, adaptability, and unpredictability.

Systems thinking—defined by P.M. Senge as "destroying the illusion that the world is created of separate unrelated forces"—can transform and advance health system development, intervention design, implementation, and outcomes. Paradigms are patterns of thinking and doing. Particular paradigms can become so embedded in our way of thinking that we may not stop to examine their appropriateness to the situation in which we are applying them. We live in an age where linear cause-and-effect paradigms and compartmentalized approaches to health and international development rule.

These paradigms are not inherently good or bad independent of the way in which they are applied. Many of the technological and scientific advances of modern times have arisen from the application of such approaches. Moreover, as knowledge builds upon preceding knowledge, the success rate of technological innovations has been more exponential than linear. Success is a powerful reinforcer of the paradigms that bring it about, as our instinct is to repeat the approach that brought us success.

However, we also live in a world where global health actors are interconnected and have the freedom to act and respond to stimuli and events in ways that are not necessarily predictable. This is a world of complex adaptive systems. In such a world, the fact that a particular paradigm brings success in one area does not mean that it will bring success in all areas. Well-meaning efforts to deliver proven interventions to scale or to respond to different problems have stumbled over the inappropriate application of linear quick-fixes that failed to account for the complex interrelationships of agents and the context of the situation to which the "fix" was applied.

A problem or an intervention in such a system is like a chair in a room with many other chairs all connected with strings that require careful observation over time to detect. A superficial glance will miss many if not all of these sometimes-near-invisible strings. Without taking the time to carefully examine and understand how the strings link the chairs, what looks like a simple and reasonable effort to change the position of one chair sets all the chairs in the room moving in unpredictable ways, creating the intended but also unintended effects. Some of these unintended effects can be chaotic or even catastrophic. To achieve any reasonable success in rearranging the chairs requires thinking that recognizes and is willing to deal with complexity, unpredictability, and paradox; and it requires an investment of time to understand as much of the interconnectivity as possible to inform how to move the chairs correctly before starting to move them. It is also important to be dynamic—observing these connections as the chairs are moving. Even when you think you have understood, once you start moving the chairs, the results may reveal that you missed.

This type of thinking recognizes that cause and effect are not necessarily directly related and that their relationship may be influenced by time, space, and many other confounding variables. Failure to understand these relationships can result in catastrophic consequences for global health. As an old nursery rhyme goes: *"For the want of a nail the shoe was lost, for the want of a shoe the horse was lost, for the want of a horse the rider was lost, for the want of a rider the battle was lost, and all for the want of a horse-shoe nail."*

The complex health systems we rely on today require adaptation and variation on our part, as opposed to continued efforts to make the systems fit age-old linear paradigms that are no longer effective. We must devise approaches that allow widespread application of systems thinking to transform health for the future.

Irene A. Agyepong is a part-time Lecturer at the University of Ghana who was formerly Regional Director of the Ghana Health Service, Prof. Prince Claus Chair in Development and Equity at Utrecht University, and Chair of Health Systems Global.

Chapter 4

Leadership for Health Equity

RECEP AKDAG

> Financing and delivering universal health care is the one change most needed in the world for better health and it can be accomplished.

Humanity has made rapid scientific and medical advances, but for those concerned with equity and the dignity of life, it can appear that our political structures have advanced at a slower pace. Going forward, I believe the most important contribution I can make is to provide an example of bringing about transformative change and to emphasize that universal health coverage should be the health sector's ultimate goal. To accomplish this goal through sustainable reform, the entire health system needs to be addressed.

As Turkey's minister of health for more than 10 years, I oversaw a transformation that radically changed the way health-care services were provided in my country. Our government created one generous single-payer health insurance scheme for all, protecting the poor. We opened all the hospitals to the public, established a new family medicine system, expanded emergency transport to rural areas, and built up resources equally throughout the country. In short, we created an accessible and affordable system that provided equity. We improved health status, decreased catastrophic health expenditures, and increased satisfaction in health services. At every turn, I faced opposition from various private interest groups who exploited the old system and from rival political parties. I had no particular training for dealing with this kind of challenge; I was not at that time a health policy expert. Instead, I relied on my experiences as a practicing physician in pediatrics.

While I was a medical student, I realized that some professors and specialists favored a small number of patients, often neglecting the rest. When I understood the reason for this disparity, I became saddened by the status quo of health care in Turkey. These doctors had private offices, in addition to their jobs at public hospitals, and they favored the patients who would pay for their private services. Fighting against this unfair practice was a battle that would last most of my career, but it was the key to reducing out-of-pocket and catastrophic health expenditures.

When I became a resident of pediatrics in 1986, the attending mothers—whose children were admitted to the hospital as inpatients—slept on the concrete floor, mostly on cardboard mats. This was often for days, and sometimes for weeks. I share this to highlight the general attitude that existed toward patients, their families, and particularly the poor. I remember a father who came to me and begged: "Please Doctor, you know my baby passed away. They won't give me my baby until I pay the bill." How shocking that the hospital had taken the dead body of this father's child hostage! I informed my professor, but he was also powerless to act against the system. It was a common practice in hospital management those days. From time to time, live patients were also kept, and employees were expected to guard them until their relatives could gather enough money to purchase their release. My first act as Turkey's minister of health was to publicly declare that significant penalties would result if the ministry discovered anyone persisting in this practice. The announcement alone helped propel my country toward deeper reforms.

Throughout my time as minister of health, the public trust was my protective shield in helping implement the transformation plan that was supported by the prime minister and the cabinet. As public support grew, my ability to help achieve substantive and lasting reforms increased as well. I used a two-pronged approach, concurrently implementing immediate changes in the most urgent cases, and pursuing comprehensive long-term strategies. Deep-rooted changes are crucial to create a sustainable transformation as they increase the public's faith in reform efforts.

As a leader, it was not my position or my expertise that shaped the direction I pushed for in making changes. Instead, it was my experience of weakness, of powerlessness, and of great sadness in the face of real and persistent pain that guaranteed I would devote everything I could to making a transformation. Today, Turkey has a very simple and comprehensive system. We provide a generous benefit package, which covers all expenses. It is the same package for all citizens, and all services are open for use by the public. It is radical in its simplicity, and simple in its motivations.

Recep Akdag is a researcher, pediatrician, and parliamentarian who formerly served as Turkey's Minister of Health from 2002 to 2013.

Chapter 5

Why Universal Health Coverage?

SUDHIR ANAND

Universal health coverage advances both health and justice in the world.

Health is critically important for two reasons: it is directly constitutive of a person's well-being, and it enables a person to function as an agent—that is, to pursue the various goals and projects in life that she has reason to value. This view deploys the notion of *health* as "well-functioning," but it is not grounded in notions of economic welfare that are based on utility or income. It is, rather, an agency-centered view of a person, for whom ill-health reduces the full scope of human agency. In the terminology of Amartya Sen, health contributes to a person's capability to function—to choose the life she has reason to value. If we see health in this way, then impairments to health constrain what people can do or be—which restricts both their well-being and their agency.

A person's long-term health and longevity are influenced by many factors, including health care and various socioeconomic, environmental, and behavioral determinants. But access to health care is also crucial in dealing with short-term illness, pain, and suffering—conditions that can affect a person's capability to function. Health care is thus central in both promoting health and responding to ill-health.

The consequence of people being denied access to health care, or it not being available, can be grave—for a person's capability to function and possibly even to survive. In such situations, the lack of health coverage is likely to be regarded as a social injustice. But how, in principle, should we characterize justice in health and health care? All approaches to justice essentially invoke impartiality, fairness, or equity in some form or other.

Sen, through appeal to a (Smithian) "impartial spectator" and a process of "public reasoning," is able to comment on national and global justice in a variety of different contexts. For example, Sen discusses the injustices involved in the non-availability of cheap (generic) drugs for poor people suffering from HIV/AIDS in developing countries; the absence of medical facilities in parts of Africa and Asia; the lack of universal health coverage in most countries in the world; and the fact of life expectancy at birth in some countries being less than *half* that in other countries.

The nature of impartiality involved is different in John Rawls's theory of "justice as fairness." Impartiality is "closed" in Rawls's "original position," whereas it is "open" in Sen's use of the impartial observer with a view, as it were, "from everywhere." Rawls's consideration of justice is limited to the sovereign- or nation-state (in a "fair system of cooperation"), and thus does not permit assessment of global injustice.

Within a sovereign state, however, we can invoke Rawls's device of impartiality (albeit closed) through his "veil of ignorance" in the original position. Behind the veil of ignorance, I do not know who I will turn out to be—and what serious illness or health problem I might face, which could require varying degrees of medical attention. In the imagined uncertainty of this original position, the institutional arrangement for health care that I am likely to favor in my nation-state is one that ensures health coverage for *all*—*universal* health coverage.

In discussing health care, an appeal to equity can also take the form that every person should be treated *equally* in response to their *need* for health care. Equity demands that people who are the same in relevant respects—in this case, have the same need for health care—are treated in a similar way: equals should be treated alike. This is the defining characteristic of what is sometimes called "horizontal equity" in the economics literature. Horizontal equity is often contrasted with "vertical equity," which requires treating relevantly different people in a different way. Different people may have different medical conditions and, therefore, different health-care needs. Vertical equity requires that people with greater health-care needs are provided with correspondingly greater health care.

I have tried here to argue the case for universal health coverage—both at the national and global level. Universal health coverage simply means that everyone who needs health care receives it. Health is among the most important conditions of human life: it directly affects a person's well-being and is a prerequisite for the person to function as an agent. The provision of universal health coverage to protect and improve people's health will be a significant contribution in advancing both health and justice in the world.

Sudhir Anand is a Professor of Economics at the University of Oxford and a Visiting Professor of Global Health and Social Medicine at Harvard Medical School.

Chapter 6

Governance and Leadership for Health

MICHELLE BACHELET

Policy must cross borders and barriers to ensure health equity for all.

Health and well-being are unquestionably linked to all spheres of society and cross national boundaries. To understand the change most needed in the world for achieving a shared future of better health, we must look to the driving forces that will affect health in the next 50 years. Over the next decades, we will live increasingly longer lives. Advances of medicine, robotics, and other innovations will reduce disabilities and extend possibilities for healthy and productive life and aging. Health and survival of humankind will be increasingly challenged by global planetary threats such as climate change, ozone depletion, desertification, biodiversity loss, and resource scarcity. These threats will be exacerbated by increasing population, longevity, and rising demands for consumption that cannot be met with our current resources. An additional challenge is growing urbanization. By 2050, 70% of the world's population will reside in cities, many in burgeoning megacities. The revolution in communication technology will continue. Society will be more informed, connected, and interdependent, and more demanding of responsiveness and accountability from governments.

Advances in science and technology will provide opportunities to increase the prediction, prevention, and treatment of disease and to improve health at a scale never seen before. However, the main challenge will be ensuring that these advances are provided equitably with measures for population technology transfer and fair benefit sharing to ensure access to health for all, with the most vulnerable first.

Undoubtedly, these driving forces will generate numerous challenges to be faced at all levels. The question is then: what type of global and national governance and leadership is critical to understand and address the health challenges of the next 50 years?

I believe that in order to address all of these challenges, global governance will need to transcend national and sectoral boundaries. As determinants of well-being shift beyond the control of individual countries, global policies will need to align and integrate to support global social, environmental, and health development challenges. Resource scarcities will need to be globally managed, and equality and solidarity must be systematically embedded in global governance. This encompasses revaluing distributional measures of well-being and environmental renewal in economic planning; encouraging ethical decision-making on technology; rethinking the balance between shareholder and stakeholder accountability; and ensuring universal coverage of benefits.

The development of new Sustainable Development Goals (SDGs) provides an opportunity to embrace these globally shared challenges. Within health, the proposed goal of achieving universal health coverage would certainly bring a greater focus to the equitable distribution of access to health, with the advantage of it being relevant for all countries, rich and poor. At the same time, it would bring attention to a set of system-level constraints that need to be addressed and the priorities that must be set to scale up access to quality health services with financial protection for all. Addressing these unprecedented challenges over the next 50 years will also require a health response with a gender lens. There is no better investment that the world can make to extend democracy, justice, and economic growth than investing in girls and women. We can no longer afford to waste the potential of half the world's population.

National leadership is critical to face health challenges. Governments will need to move toward higher levels of solidarity, collaboration, and inclusion, overcoming isolation, individualism, and exclusion. The type of leadership required includes putting people at the center of all policies, making a commitment to solidarity and equality, and having the ability to oversee and engage in complexity. National leaders must be able to form connections from local to global health; to think strategically, listen to people, facilitate, and steer national processes that lead to better and more equitable health; and to mobilize multiple actors within their countries to achieve health goals. The contribution of the private sector is also critical. Companies will have to better balance private shareholder interests, taking a longer view of returns, to cooperate with the state and society to improve health and health equity within their countries.

Development and health in particular can no longer be understood as a summative of private goods, with access based on individual ability to pay. Instead, they must be viewed as global public goods, governed by shared responsibility, which is embraced by global and national leaders alike. A future of collective well-being is possible and within reach. We can wield our unique abilities to embrace change and innovate, soaring past boundaries to take us to a shared future of sustained health.

Michelle Bachelet is President of the Republic of Chile and former Executive Director of the United Nations Entity for Gender Equality and the Empowerment of Women (UN Women).

Chapter 7

Prioritizing Vulnerable Populations

JOYCE BANDA

To improve health, we must address the barriers facing the most vulnerable and marginalized populations, with a particular focus on women and children.

If health is to be advanced, we need to measure leaders not by the armies they command, or by the size of their nation's economy, but by the improvements they make in the lives of their country's most vulnerable populations. These are the people living on the margins of socioeconomic, political, and cultural systems. More often than not, these are women and children. Leaders should be measured by their commitment to make this world a better place for *all* to live in, and by the efforts they make to turn the "period of pregnancy" from being a period of anxiety to a time of excitement and hope. By caring for the most vulnerable, especially poor women and children, we can lay the foundation for global health, peace, and prosperity.

As president of Malawi, I made the well-being of women and children a national priority. My commitment to this issue began years earlier, in my own childhood. Though my family lived in a town, I spent every weekend in my grandmother's village, where I had a good friend named Chrissie. Chrissie was one of the brightest students in the village school, and we were both selected to attend the best secondary school for girls in Malawi. Sadly, Chrissie had to drop out of school after her first term because her parents could not afford the six-dollar school fee.

She returned to the village, where she married and had six children. She has lived in poverty ever since.

What happened to Chrissie is unjust and unacceptable. But what is most tragic is that there are many Chrissies in the world. Our hopes for a healthy future are bound up with the lives of people like Chrissie and her children. Girls who do not finish school are forced into early marriages and have children at a tender age. They are at high risk for maternal deaths and complications and their children are more likely to remain poor. Lack of basic health services, including family planning, takes a devastating toll on the health of women and children, which undercuts productivity and economic development.

However, there is hope. The vicious cycle can be broken. To confront the challenges of the twenty-first century—global health, sustainable development, climate change—we have to redefine our approach as we seek to address the many problems facing women and girls. All the problems that they are grappling with emanate from their lack of economic empowerment, which is key not only to women's emancipation but also to socioeconomic development and the attainment of the Millennium Development Goals that sadly have eluded many developing countries. We have to take a holistic approach that focuses on incomes, girls' education, and women's health, rights, and participation in decision-making processes and circles. When families have adequate income, they are able to send their female children to school and support them. They can also access good health care and meet other essentials of better living.

Investing in women's health pays enormous dividends. If a young woman has access to sexual and reproductive health services, she stays in school longer, gets married later, has fewer and healthier children, and has more opportunities to participate in economic and civic life.

Healthy, educated citizens are an essential foundation of a vibrant economy, which is a precursor to peace. This is not news, and yet there are very few countries—rich or poor—in which the health and well-being of vulnerable women and children are a national priority. That must change. And it will only change if leaders are held accountable to their most vulnerable citizens.

As former president of Malawi and now as a member of the Global Leaders Council for Reproductive Health, I have fought for girls' education, maternal and child health, and women's empowerment. I can point to many achievements on those fronts of which I am proud. But looking back, this is how I measure the success of my tenure in office: today there is a school—an excellent, free secondary school—in the village where Chrissie lives.

Joyce Banda is the former President of the Republic of Malawi and a member of the Global Leaders Council for Reproductive Health.

Chapter 8

The New Health Journalism

JULIA BELLUZ

Upheaval in the media is not necessarily a bad thing for health reporting; journalists can now have a greater impact on public health than ever before.

Most people who read health journalism with a critical gaze would say it's in bad shape. For evidence, look no further than your local newspaper (if one still exists) or open your favorite website and learn about "the 10 ways to bust your belly fat for good." Coffee, you surely know by now, will help you live longer on Monday and kill you quicker by the weekend.

It is usually assumed that this state of affairs is linked to the collapse of media as we knew it. Gone are the days when science desks were staples of newsrooms and journalists had time to read the studies that they reported on or call their best sources. Those pseudoscientific examples of health journalism, the argument goes, are nothing more than side effects of a traditional media that has fallen ill. The oft-cited causes of the disease: digital upheaval, a decline in advertising revenue, and the death knell of global financial crisis.

The news business can be gloomy but the prognosis for health reporting matters for three reasons. First, people barely follow their doctor's prescriptions, yet they will bet their health and dollars on whatever miracle cure is being touted in the media. This is as true for Dr. Oz's weight-loss wonders in America as it is for cricket players who promote the polio vaccine in Pakistan. Second, decision-makers, like politicians, policymakers, and even doctors, rely on journalists to tell them what's new and important in the world of medicine and health research. When journalists get it wrong, their work can have a harmful, reverberating impact. Third, health care is a business like any other and it needs to be kept accountable. The fourth estate, it should be clear by now, is not only a pillar of a functioning democracy; it's a pillar of public health.

While this is no doubt the case, the idea that health journalism is at its end stages is no longer true. We are in the midst of a journalism revolution, and if harnessed for public health, the press can have a greater positive impact than ever before. New media ventures such as *Vox* and *FiveThirtyEight* use the endless space afforded by the Internet to explain the news in a more nuanced and research-driven manner than print media—with its limited real estate—ever could. Stories link back to primary sources and studies so that readers can immediately verify or follow up as part of their news-consuming experience.

At Vox, we link news updates in "storystreams" so audiences can see how reporting developed over time. "Card stacks" answer readers' most basic questions so they have more entry points to important stories. We are no longer confined by the artificial limits of daily print deadlines; instead, we post quickly and develop our coverage as we learn more. When you think about online news this way, anxieties about too much speed and reactivity dissipate. Instead, journalists can now report the news and new research as they were meant to—in an iterative and contextualized manner that actually reflects current events and science as they evolve.

The digital revolution in media has also given rise to a cadre of science-oriented blogs like Retraction Watch, Science-Based Medicine, and Bad Science. They publish more frequently than traditional beat reporters, correcting the record, illuminating health research, and holding pseudoscience opinion-leaders or decision-makers to account. In addition to speaking directly to their sizable audiences, their work is picked up by mainstream media or they are called upon as sources, elevating the discourse about science along the way.

Many of these bloggers came from academia and would have never had a voice beyond the Ivory Tower. Now, they do, as the gap between research and journalism shrinks.

This new direction includes reporting on and using "big data" for journalism. Every day, the amount of data we produce grows, and journalists have more at their disposal to learn about themselves and the world. We can also measure the scope and impact of our work more easily and precisely than we ever could previously. We can quantify which health topics we reported on, which ones we ignored, and how that compares with other important factors such as public investment in research and disease burden.

With potential come pitfalls. More information means more *bad* information. Big data cannot replace old-fashioned journalistic inquiry. But in this time of media transition, health journalists need to keep their eyes on the possibilities. We need to remember that, whether we like it or not, our stories are often used as medicine by readers. We need to publish with the care and deliberateness of a doctor writing a prescription and use all the new tools at our disposal to make sure it's a prescription that will actually help. Billions of people are counting on us.

Julia Belluz is a National Magazine Award-winning journalist focused on medicine and public health at Vox.com and a former MIT Knight Science Journalism Fellow.

Chapter 9

Vaccines—Accelerating Access for All

SETH BERKLEY

The last 20 years have seen an acceleration of new vaccines, which has expanded our ability to prevent disease before it hurts us.

Knowledge of how infectious disease can be prevented through intentional exposure to the disease dates back to as far as the ancient Egyptians. Yet, it wasn't until around 200 years ago that the era of vaccination truly began. After observing that milkmaids never seemed to suffer the scourge of smallpox, pioneer Edward Jenner hypothesized that they were being afforded some form of protection from the cows that they milked. Convinced of his theory, in 1796 Jenner deliberately gave cowpox, a bovine virus similar to smallpox, to an 8-year-old boy and 22 others in the hope of protecting them from human smallpox. It worked! Naming his technique *vaccination*—after "vacca," the Latin word for cow—he began a revolution that continues to this day. At its peak, smallpox killed two million people a year and meant disability for millions more who survived. By 1977, smallpox had been completely eradicated through what some say was the greatest public health success ever.

Despite their huge success with smallpox, only a dozen vaccines were developed in the 150 years after Jenner's groundbreaking work because of the limitations of primitive scientific techniques. Recently, however, thanks to modern laboratory methods and improved technology, there has been an explosion in development, and over 50 new vaccines have been produced. A polio vaccine was discovered in the 1950s, and the disease is now teetering on the verge of eradication, with only a few hundred cases still occurring in the world. Today, the World Health Organization (WHO) recommends 11 vaccines for every child—diphtheria, pertussis, tetanus, polio, *Haemophilus influenzae* type b (Hib), hepatitis B (hepB), measles, rubella, BCG (against tuberculosis), pneumococcal, rotavirus—as well as HPV for all adolescents. Other vaccines are recommended for particular geographic areas. In wealthy developed countries with high vaccine coverage, these diseases mostly have disappeared.

In the developing world, this has not been the case. In 1975, less than 5% of children in developing countries received the six basic vaccines then recommended. A concerted effort has changed that; in 2013 as many as 83% of children worldwide received these six vaccines—although this average hides the disparities. In developing countries, more than 22 million children, or 26%, do not receive these basic vaccines. Furthermore, less than 5% receive the 11 vaccines currently recommended for global use by WHO. Yet these powerful new vaccines target the most common causes of diarrhea and pneumonia—rotavirus and pneumococcal—the two largest killers of children worldwide. Efforts to provide access to these new vaccines through my organization, Gavi, the Vaccine Alliance, are accelerating; it is estimated that by 2020 more than half the children in the world will be fully covered by the 11 recommended vaccines.

Access is partially a result of financial limitations, which we try to ameliorate by subsidizing vaccine purchases in low-income countries. But developing countries are also constrained by their health systems infrastructure. Use of new tools such as digital information systems, supply chain modernization, geographical information systems, and better human resource management has been allowing countries to leapfrog into much higher performing systems, thereby enabling dramatic increases in access to vaccines and other vital health interventions.

Newer vaccines have also moved us from prevention of traditional childhood infectious diseases to addressing infectious causes of chronic diseases, such as cancer. Today we are rolling out vaccines against infections implicated in two common cancers: liver cancer (hepB) and cervical cancer (HPV). Many other cancers are already known to have infectious antecedents, such as helicobacter pylori and stomach cancer, Epstein-Barr virus and lymphoma, and human T-lymphotropic virus (HTLV) and leukemia. Today more than 30% of cancers in Africa have known infectious antecedents as opposed to about less than 10% in developed countries. With further investigations, this number will likely increase. Many other chronic diseases, such as type 1 diabetes, inflammatory bowel disease, and some forms of arthritis, have characteristics that suggest that infection may play some type of role. As a result, vaccines may be developed in the future to prevent many of these diseases.

Adding to this optimism, science is now creating new paradigms to create vaccines for many of the more difficult agents, where correlates of protection are poorly defined and where pathogens evade standard immunologic detection or have extensive variability and adaptability. Such infectious diseases include HIV, hepatitis C, malaria, and tuberculosis, which have thus far challenged traditional vaccinology. By using new mechanisms of rational vaccine development, similar to those currently used in drug development, scientists are now redefining what is possible.

The fact is our ability to protect people from disease, through the provision of safe and effective vaccines, will only continue to rise. This fills me with great hope. While we have already seen the enormous public health benefits of existing vaccines, we are still only just beginning to understand the economic and social advances that accompany them. As technology continues to improve, we appear set to enter into a transformational renaissance of even more powerful disease prevention.

Seth Berkley is the CEO of Gavi, the Vaccine Alliance, and founder and former President and CEO of the International AIDS Vaccine Initiative.

Chapter 10

Improving Health by Addressing Poverty

ELA BHATT

The harsh realities of poverty are too often lost on health implementers; a community-minded approach is needed for effective change.

In a country where a majority of the population is poor, improving the health of its people is inextricably linked to addressing the root causes and consequences of poverty. Poverty has a tendency to interfere with our neat notions of health care. If everyone had access to nutritious foods, safe drinking water, clean air, and proper sewage disposal, the number of diseases in the world would possibly halve. Yet, these universal panaceas are elusive in the daily lives of the poor. Strenuous manual work for long hours, under harsh conditions, and for a meager daily wage, is the reality for most of the working poor. Keeping these realities in mind when looking at health-care solutions forces us to alter and broaden our vision.

Advising a woman in rural Gujarat, India, that boiling water will significantly cut down her risk of infection is not enough. It is equally important to make sure she has the ability to do so. This means that our definition of health care must also include providing access to clean water and adequate fuel to boil that water. Similarly, the treatment for common digestive-tract diseases lies as much in access to toilets and a functioning sewage system as it does in medicines and rehydration.

By looking at the different jobs upon which a country's economy is built, one can see the occupational health hazards that its people face. In India, salt workers suffer from eye, lung, and skin ailments; agricultural workers suffer the effects of chemicals and pesticides; cart pullers and head-loaders commonly miscarry when pregnant; tobacco workers and their children bear the consequences of nicotine poisoning. In such cases, disease prevention not only involves protective equipment, but it also requires providing day care, ergonomic technology, and, above all, social security and strengthened labor laws.

A network of well-equipped hospitals and primary health clinics dispensing low-cost medicines are indeed vital to curative care. Equally vital are the mobile health-care workers who live in the community, treat basic ailments, deliver babies, immunize children, and become a source of knowledge about the workings of the body and the kind of environment in which it thrives. In poor countries, investing in buildings and infrastructure is important, but it is also capital intensive; investing in people, on the other hand, is relatively economical, and it sets in motion a change in society with far-reaching, long-lasting effect.

In my view, the root causes and consequences of poverty and exploitation are just as important for health as caring for particular maladies after they occur. We must take this broader view and focus our efforts on this basis.

Ela Bhatt is Founder of the Self Employed Women's Association of India and a member of The Elders.

Chapter 11

Biosocial Education for All

AGNES BINAGWAHO

To improve health, we should introduce biosocial analysis training into formal education around the world.

The current gap in equitable access to the many medical and scientific advances of recent decades is troubling. We have what it takes to achieve equity, but real progress is lagging far behind. If we wish to fulfill the human right to health and improve population well-being, we need to make health the concern of each and every citizen through our education systems. To achieve this, we must formally introduce the notion that reaching local and global health objectives is the responsibility of every person, household, village, neighborhood, city, and country.

To improve global health, I think we need to systematically integrate the biosocial aspects of medicine and health care into all national education systems. When the social aspects of health problems faced by patients and families are better understood, our communities and clinicians will be able to offer better support and care. Such integration through all education systems—formal, informal, and vocational training—will expose students around the world to a broad understanding of how people fall ill, and how people get better. In this way, health professionals will broaden their analytical skill set, develop a more nuanced comprehension of ethics, and bolster their problem-solving abilities.

This need not be limited to medical training. Requiring this integration in primary and secondary schools will allow young people to learn early on that health and well-being are affected by more than what is understood to be the traditional health sector. Health is also affected by its social determinants—food security, income, stress, housing, and infrastructure. At 7 years old, most children will begin to understand the moral notions of good and bad, of justice and injustice, of social environment, and of health and sickness. As such, even at the primary education level, we have an opportunity to start positively shaping a child's views on what it means and what it takes to be healthy—a mindset that can be reinforced throughout the remainder of his or her education.

The curricula for such training would certainly be deepened each year as students advance, and specific adaptations would be made for a community's culture, history, and family practices. By starting young, these concepts would already be familiar, and the curricula would be designed to build upon the lessons learned in previous years.

The approach would be integrated into graduate programs and higher education. For example, students pursuing an advanced degree would take a course on the biosocial and health aspects of their field of study. Dissertations in fields commonly considered to be unrelated to health would include at least a paragraph analyzing how the subject is important for individual or population health using a biosocial analysis. This would inevitably bring continuous new knowledge to improve health for all of humanity. Moreover, for students in fields with a more direct overlap with health care—like medicine, education, architecture, or any of the social sciences—a full course on biosocial analysis and how each student's work directly impacts the majority of the social determinants of health would be necessary.

I offer an out-of-the-box case: among the most respected jobs in the world is the ship captain. This is a field for which training is regarded as being fairly distant from health, is it not? But the actions of ship captains and their crews can indeed have implications for population well-being. For instance, ships can take on ballast water in one location and let it off on arrival elsewhere (often very far away). This method can easily transport non-native species that are dangerous to human health. If there were a lifelong focus in education on biosocial analysis, trainees who wish to work in such industries would have a heightened awareness of these health issues and they could take the necessary precautions. Of course this is just one illustration of many.

Continuous biosocial education and training would foster a culture driven to examine the impact of social determinants of health, across all sectors, and equip all professionals to propose or contribute to solutions for key global and local challenges. Knowing that the underlying cause of 90% of the barriers to good health are beyond the confines of the traditional "health sector" will help revolutionize efforts toward improving it.

In one generation, this new model of education would equip professionals, across all ages and disciplines, with an understanding of the social determinants of health, and it would help foster the thinking and motivation needed to fulfill the right to health. This could be achieved through a United Nations General Assembly declaration, like the one adopted on HIV/AIDS. Biosocial education will improve our ability to respect the dignity, the participation, and the entitlement to the right to health of all fellow humans. In this way, our world will be more prepared than ever before to understand and protect health for the generations to come.

Agnes Binagwaho is the Minister of Health of Rwanda, Senior Lecturer of Global Health and Social Medicine at Harvard Medical School, and Clinical Professor of Pediatrics at Dartmouth College.

Chapter 12

City Leadership on Climate Change

MICHAEL BLOOMBERG

By fighting climate change, we improve public health immediately.

Some of the most exciting developments in public health are happening in the world's cities—and few have greater potential to improve our lives than city-led efforts to confront climate change.

This is true for two reasons. The first is that, if we do nothing to mitigate climate change, we run terrible public health risks. It is expected that in some parts of the world, rising temperatures will make it too hot and humid to safely be outside for parts of the year and cause some infectious diseases to spread more rapidly; crop losses will drive up food prices, threaten supplies, and cause hunger; and more lives will be lost as sea levels rise and extreme weather becomes more frequent. Some of the worst consequences will be felt in developing countries, where weak infrastructure and lack of access to medical resources will compound the health risks facing vulnerable populations.

The second reason is that the steps cities take to combat climate change will not only help avoid such a future, but they will also improve public health today. The link between climate change action and public health improvements could not be clearer. Some of the major sources of carbon emissions that cause climate change—like power plants, buildings, and automobiles—also contribute to serious and avoidable health problems. By focusing on these sources in cities, where the world's population and carbon emissions are concentrated, we can make major progress in the fight against climate change, while also improving the health of the world's people.

For instance, in New York City, buildings are the largest source of both carbon emissions and air pollution. Transitioning buildings to cleaner-burning heating fuels helped reduce the city's carbon emissions by 19% in just six years, while also reducing the particulate matter that contributes to asthma and other respiratory ailments. Today, New York City's air is cleaner than it has been in more than 50 years—a key reason life expectancy in the city increased nearly three years during my time as mayor, far outpacing the national increase.

In addition to making buildings greener and more efficient, cities around the world are also investing in smarter transportation systems as a way of reducing their carbon footprint and air pollution. By implementing bus rapid transit, making streets safer for pedestrians and cyclists, and adding public bike-sharing programs, cities are lowering emissions by keeping cars off the road. Such efforts reduce health problems from air pollution as well as traffic deaths and injuries. Low-carbon public transportation systems, because they encourage mobility, can also help prevent obesity and the health problems it causes, like heart disease and diabetes.

Concerns about public health can galvanize actions that also help mitigate climate change. We've seen this in the United States where my foundation has been working with the Sierra Club on the Beyond Coal campaign to shut coal-fired power plants and keep new ones from opening. Burning coal is the single largest source of carbon emissions in the country, and it also takes a terrible toll on public health. Emissions from coal-fired power plants in the United States contribute to 13,000 deaths every year and sicken tens of thousands of people.

Beyond Coal has been very successful in gathering local support for coal plant closures, in large part because people don't want to be near power plants that cause sickness and death. To date, Beyond Coal has helped reduce the country's total coal inventory by more than a third—which will prevent some 5,000 deaths and 72,000 asthma attacks a year, while also saving $2 billion annually in health-care costs. In addition, the reduction in coal power, driven by plant closures, is a major reason why US carbon emissions have dropped to their lowest levels in 20 years.

Public health concerns are helping drive local climate action elsewhere in the world as well. For example, in China—the world's largest carbon emitter—the alarming prevalence of health problems caused by air pollution has led local governments to take action, reducing both pollution and carbon emissions. Meanwhile, in India, the city of Delhi addressed public health concerns about air pollution by switching its taxis and buses to natural gas, which also reduces carbon emissions.

By taking steps like these, cities are leading the way in combating the long-term effects of climate change. In doing so, they are also achieving major public health victories that benefit people today. With the majority of the world's population living in cities for the first time—and 75% expected to be city dwellers by 2050—encouraging cities to invest in sustainability is one of our greatest opportunities to improve lives.

Michael Bloomberg is the founder of Bloomberg LP and Bloomberg Philanthropies, UN Special Envoy for Cities and Climate Change, and former Mayor of New York City from 2002 to 2013.

Chapter 13

Health Is Not Alone

ALBINA DU BOISROUVRAY

Achieving better health means addressing other basic human needs.

Poverty is not simply a lack of money; it is a debilitating state of deprivation—a lack of material and intangible tools—that thwarts one's ability to attain and sustain good health, even when medical services are available. With that in mind, having access to health care is irrelevant in the absence of food, shelter, income, education, and life skills. All of these factors, together, are what defines good health.

In 1986, my son died in a tragic accident. François-Xavier Bagnoud had been an alpine helicopter rescue pilot; he had, from childhood, a passion for rescuing people. To honor his memory, I wanted to do what I could do to rescue children orphaned by HIV/AIDS from falling into a never-ending, downward spiral of deprivation. The Association François-Xavier Bagnoud (AFXB), the organization I set up 25 years ago, pioneered a family- and community-based approach to improving global health and eradicating poverty. The approach centers on providing unconditional short-term support for basic needs, all part of a larger investment in poor people's ability to achieve and *sustain* good health and well-being over the long term.

In 1989, the fashionable approach to poverty eradication was a single-minded focus on micro-credit: lend money to poor people—especially women—to start a self-sustaining business. I soon realized, however, that people living in extreme unremitting poverty would never be able to repay the money—not unless they were to kill off their businesses in the process.

A better approach is to recognize the inextricable links between human rights and human health, the relationship articulated best by the late World Health Organization leader Jonathan Mann. He argued that only by promoting human rights could public health policies be both effective and sustainable. A woman who does not have the right to refuse sex with a husband infected with HIV will probably die, having given birth to infected children who will, in turn, become orphans. In this rather stark example, both human rights and public health have been done a disservice in turn.

And so was born the FXBVillage methodology to emphasize the link between health and human rights. Our first FXBVillage in Uganda initially focused on four drivers of poverty eradication: we repaired houses and built new ones; we helped the community grow its own food; we provided health care, including psychological counseling; and we offered families and communities education, including training in personal finances.

But we needed to take Dr. Mann's thinking further. The danger of an approach based solely on the provision of basic needs is that it fails to equip people with the capabilities they need to sustain their own well-being. So, FXBVillages now include a fifth driver—a business—that will, within three years, not only provide a living for the family involved, but also generate enough surplus to continue to provide housing, health care, nutrition, and education. This final driver delivers a truly workable route to a self-sustaining community. We have found that after three years, financial support can be safely withdrawn.

One of many examples of how the model has promoted lasting health is offered in the person of Nite, a Ugandan woman who was HIV-positive and destitute 10 years ago. In 1995, she was given one cow. A decade later she had three cows, two pigs, and some chickens, as well as land on which she is growing pineapples and coffee and has built a house. Relieved of her distressed state and equipped to advocate for her rights, Nite gained confidence and the capacity to meet her health needs and generate enough income to put all her children through school.

Two of her children later went on to university and one found gainful employment abroad. Time-limited support with few strings attached afforded Nite the breathing room, along with the tools and conditions, essential for cultivating good health and improving her family's social status, thus setting a new path for future generations. She remains alive and well today.

Our experience proves that sustainable health and well-being requires opportunity alongside material conditions. This is why this approach has won the endorsement of acclaimed Nobel Laureate Amartya Sen and countless others who work with and support FXBVillages around the world.

The world pays insufficient attention to the biggest underlying cause of poor health: poverty. For global health to be realized, policymakers, health-care providers, and well-meaning people with influence must challenge traditional approaches, eschew myopic development, and commit to tackling health problems holistically. Health is not the singular or end-all, be-all goal, but rather part of an intricate set of basic human needs, rights, and capabilities that demand our creative and concerted attention. We need to think holistically and outside the box to provide all of them to everyone.

Albina du Boisrouvray is the Founder of Association François-Xavier Bagnoud, FXB Foundation, and FXB International.

Chapter 14

Education First

IRINA BOKOVA

Education is a health multiplier that is essential for disease prevention and better health outcomes.

"I wish I had gone to school because if you don't know how to read and write, it is difficult to educate your children. A woman will better understand the explanation given to her by a nurse when she goes for maternal consultations, and this is useful for any mother for her children's fate." These words of Ms. Leza Souley, of Niger, say it all.

Education is a health multiplier and is essential for disease prevention and better health outcomes. As shown in UNESCO's most recent Education for All Global Monitoring Report, education saves millions of lives every year, it prevents and contains disease, and it reduces malnutrition. Educated women and men are better informed, take more preventative measures, recognize signs of illness earlier, and tend to use health-care services more often.

That said, the fact that there are 793 million illiterate adults and over 100 million girls and boys out of school throws a shadow over the health prospects of entire societies.

The power of education is especially clear for girls and women. Between 1990 and 2009, the lives of 2.1 million children under the age of 5 were saved thanks to improvements in the education of women of reproductive age. If all women completed primary education, there would be 66% fewer maternal deaths. Educated mothers are better informed about diseases, and as such, they can take preventive measures. Diarrhea is the fourth biggest killer of children worldwide; if all women in low- and lower-middle-income countries finished primary education, the incidence of diarrhea would fall by 8%, and by 30% with secondary education. The same goes for the chance of a child being immunized against diphtheria, tetanus, and whooping cough—this would increase by 43% if all women in these countries received secondary education.

Improving education is essential to reducing the incidence of infectious diseases like HIV/AIDS. It is also the key to tackling malnutrition, which is the underlying cause of more than 45% of child deaths. Likewise, ensuring that girls stay in school is one of the most effective ways to prevent child marriage. An estimated one in eight girls is married by the age of 15 in sub-Saharan Africa and South West Asia. This can lead to a lifetime of disadvantage and deprivation. Staying in school longer gives girls the confidence to make choices that avert the health risks of early births and births in quick succession. Overall, educated women also tend to have fewer children.

This list of benefits is long, yet education is far too neglected as a health intervention in itself and a means to enhance other health interventions. Today, there are still 58 million children out of primary school and 63 million adolescents out of school. The stakes are high.

I am not referring to just any form of education. To be effective, education must be inclusive for all girls and boys, regardless of their circumstances. It must be relevant, providing useful knowledge and skills for learners to protect themselves and create a healthy social and physical environment. It must be empowering and promote the human rights and dignity of every learner.

This calls for work at the legislative level to prevent discrimination and to craft policies for supporting access. It means abolishing school fees and providing incentives for parents to send their children to school. We need concerted efforts in developing national educational strategies to train teachers to promote health and sexuality education, and to create safe and gender-sensitive conditions in schools for girls. We need to work at every level, including on nutrition, to keep girls and boys in school all the way through secondary education.

This is a concern for national governments and the United Nations, but not only for them—health concerns all of society. This is why UNESCO is teaming up with the private sector to improve literacy for girls and women. For one partnership, we are promoting puberty education and menstrual hygiene management, calling on ministries of education to ensure that girls receive education about puberty, as well as access to private and safe toilets. Sharing examples of good practices, we have also identified the importance of ensuring that boys receive puberty education as well.

New vaccines and medicines carry tremendous promise for human well-being, but we need to educate people—especially girls and women—to make the most of these new opportunities. This is why the nexus between education and health must be at the heart of the post-2015 global development agenda and reflected in new development goals. As the Nobel Prize-winning activist Malala Yousafzai put it, the "best solution is education—education makes girls independent and realize they have equal rights." This is the beginning of better health.

Irina Bokova is Director-General of the United Nations Educational, Scientific and Cultural Organization (UNESCO) and former Minister of Foreign Affairs of Bulgaria.

Chapter 15

Pandemic's One-Two-Three Punch

LARRY BRILLIANT

Alongside the obvious first punch to the health of humanity from a catastrophic pandemic, there are poorly understood longer lasting second and third punches that can create unpredictable negative spirals.

The greatest challenges to global health are the three "punches" to modern civilization that a major disruptive pandemic may bring.

We all know the first punch: the toll of the sick and the dead, upwards of tens of millions could die, or even hundreds of millions or more if we extrapolate from events like the 1917 influenza pandemic. But no matter how devastating, our health systems are better prepared for this first punch than what will follow.

The second "punch" would be massive population dislocations, suspension of air, ship, and train travel, diminished world trade, famine-level shortages of goods and services, and the increased risk of failed states.

It is the third "punch," however, that we are totally unprepared for: the loss of civility, the global grieving and despair, and the "apocalyptic and post-apocalyptic" loss of hope. A pandemic of this scale could unwind the enormous gains in health and quality of life that advances in science, public health, and medical technology have given us since the end of World War II.

In working for the Skoll Global Threats Fund, my team and I helped with the science and accuracy of the movie "Contagion," trying to make a Hollywood production reflect the likely effects of a globally disruptive pandemic on a modern hyper-networked world—not the hyped nor the fantastic. No matter how careful, accurate, and understated we tried to depict the pandemic, it was impossible to escape the conclusion that modern life as we know it would be torn apart if historical pandemics were extrapolated into today's time and circumstances.

The last three decades alone have seen the emergence of three dozen or so "pandemic-potential" organisms, mostly zoonotic viruses that jumped from animals to humans. So far, some of these organisms have spread like wildfire, others have killed most of their victims, but none, thankfully, have done both. It is very important to repeat that none of the terrible recent outbreaks (e.g., SARS, MERS, Ebola, swine flu, avian flu) has had historic levels of both high transmissibility and high case fatality at the same time.

Most epidemiologists will attribute this to good luck, the fortunate spin of the genetic roulette wheel. Many will also say that is not a matter of "if" but of "when" a virus with both attributes jumps to humans. Think for a moment of a disease with the spreading capacity of smallpox or swine flu coupled with the case fatality of Ebola.

We can cope with high death rates. We can manage with high transmissibility. What we cannot overplan for is the so-called long-tail risk of the knock-on effects of a high fatality rate coupled with high transmissibility in a virus that our systems are late discovering and responding to. The devastation would dwarf either world war in its debilitating effects.

Why is this? Because of modernity, population growth, and the increased speed of travel, the second punch of a pandemic could turn the virtues of globalization and technology against us. Our connectedness, our international mobility, and our complex "just in time" supply chains for food, drugs, and key utilities would all switch from sustainers of modernity to nemeses. Our airports would close, our hospitals would be overwhelmed, our corporations unable to move goods and services around the planet, our schools unable to operate, and our health workers decimated. Our communication systems and political institutions are simply not strong enough to deal with such overwhelming and widespread overload.

The aftermath of the 2010 eruptions of the Icelandic volcano, Eyjafjallajökull, on flower-exporting African economies; the "quarantine" costs in Toronto after the 2003 SARS epidemic; the West Africa Ebola outbreak; these are just small tastes of how our interconnectedness can contribute to the unraveling of social infrastructure, fragile national economies, and the postapocalyptic vision of despair and destroyed hope.

Fortunately, we are nowhere near that inevitability yet. In the race to build a robust, sustainable, and resilient world, I think we are winning today because of early detection and early effective response to pandemic-potential organisms. Two decades ago, a pandemic-potential virus could leap from an animal to a human and not be detected for six months. If lethal viruses are given a six-month "head start," the toll could quickly reach hundreds of millions of cases. Today, as governments, foundations, academic institutions, and civil society organizations work together to build stronger institutions, the average speed of detection of an emergent virus is closer to three weeks, a world of difference.

At Skoll Global Threats Fund, we work on early detection and response, and building alliances to coordinate response to potential pandemics. Other foundations and organizations work on treatment, vaccination, policy and education, and supporting the panoply of institutional collaborations that work to limit the spread of disease. In dealing with pandemic prevention, we are, quite literally, all in this together.

Systemic threats of this kind call for systemic thinking. They require countries, global governing bodies, nonprofits, and corporations to collectively plan in advance and coordinate both epidemiological and cultural responses. We have made excellent progress in preparing for a pandemic's first punch, like stockpiling vaccines, early detection, and coordination of public health response. We have also made some progress in preparing for the economic, governance, and political dislocations that would follow. What scares me most is how we have made no progress at all in preventing the third "punch." We need to start thinking about how to limit blame, restore trust, and build hope in the face of fear and uncertainty. Only then will we be prepared against pandemics' one-two-three punch.

Larry Brilliant is Senior Advisor with the Skoll Global Threats Fund and former head of Google.org.

Chapter 16

Equality Is the Future

GRO HARLEM BRUNDTLAND

Understanding that inequality is both unacceptable and unnecessary is the first step in moving toward a healthier tomorrow.

Toward the end of the last century, as I was addressing the executive board of the World Health Organization (WHO) as a candidate for the office of Director-General, I made the point that no investments in this world yield higher socioeconomic profits than investments in people's health.

The international community had already discovered the key role of education. The time had come to apply that same focus to health. Ill health leads to poverty, and poverty breeds ill health.

There was a danger that the appalling health gaps that already existed between the rich and the poor would widen. Narrowing these gaps, both between and within states, had to be our main focus.

My main concern was that the role of health in development had for much too long been underestimated, even when human health was the true common denominator at key United Nations conferences such as Rio, Vienna, Cairo, Copenhagen, and Beijing. These meetings had also brought to the forefront the key role of reproductive health, of women in health, as well as in social and economic development.

I argued that WHO should be a catalyst for raising the status of health in international politics. Health is pivotal. Health is the core of human development. In the years since then, a lot has happened to elevate health on the global political agenda, as new partnerships have been formed and important results achieved. World history demonstrates how great the advances in health and life expectancy have been over the last hundred years, as science and new knowledge have helped us overcome a number of key challenges to health and longevity. It also shows us how democracy, participation, and broad-based economic growth have led to pivotal changes in societies and brought about improvements in people's lives and livelihoods.

Today, I want to make clear that behind it all, and as the basis for where I believe the world should be moving forward, is equity and justice. Overcoming inequality, not just in health, but in life overall, should be a top global priority. We must reduce the now growing gaps between people in different countries, and even those inhabiting the same country. It is not sufficient to deliver prevention and life-saving vaccinations or other knowledge-based interventions; we must ensure they are available to all people. We must also address the root causes of persisting health inequities, as they are also directly linked to those of other inequities that negatively affect humanity.

Inequality is rampant. It is unacceptable as well as unnecessary. This is the foremost transformative insight that will advance health.

It gives me new hope that the recent book by the French economist Thomas Piketty has helped increase global awareness and concern about the dramatic and unacceptable levels of inequality that have been developing in later decades, not least in the United States. Capitalism was supposed to "lift all boats," but instead it led to the accumulation of capital in the hands of a select few. Redistributive initiatives and expanded social programs following World War II prevented inequalities from growing, but since the early eighties this trend has been reversed because of changes in policies, and this has led to the constantly growing gaps among us at present. This alarming situation will persist unless decisive political action is taken. Progressive taxation and determined redistributive policies are urgently needed, for justice, stability, peace, and sustainable development.

The impressive knowledge that humanity has accumulated on issues of crucial importance to human health is not available to so many individuals and communities, the same ones hit the hardest by the dramatic consequences of inequality. It should let us always keep in mind how essential equality and justice are, for human progress itself.

Unless we become much more effective and determined as national and global communities to share and apply the knowledge we have acquired, unnecessary and unacceptable suffering will be the result. As poorer countries try to develop, they should be able to count on their wealthier neighbors for support. However, the most important decision that poorer countries will make as they move forward is how they choose to invest in and focus on the very basis of their prosperity—their own people.

Health and education are keys to success. So is investing in and inspiring equal opportunities for girls and women. When half of your society is being held back, how can you even hope for success?

Gro Harlem Brundtland is the Deputy Chair of The Elders, UN Special Envoy on Climate Change, former Director-General of the World Health Organization, and former Prime Minister of Norway.

Chapter 17

Prioritizing Health in Politics

FELIPE CALDERÓN

Governments must make health a real priority and express that in concrete actions and programs, but especially in budgets.

To be an effective president of a country, there is a basic rule one must follow: establish clear priorities, order them according to their importance, and then allocate energy, time, and resources proportionally toward addressing them. In the case of health care, if governments want to make it a priority and have a real impact, they'll need to show their commitment in actions and programs—but mainly in budgets.

For an ordinary person, health is clearly a priority. Strangely, not all governments feel the same way. In Mexico we have a saying: "Health comes first." I personally have seen families sacrifice everything they have and take on debts at high interest rates just to be able to pay for health services. Governments, meanwhile, spend billions on things that are ultimately far less consequential.

The house in Morelia, Mexico, where I grew up and where my mother still lives was close to many hospitals and a medical school. Every day we would see people who had traveled for days to reach the state capital from isolated villages just to see a doctor. Many of the scenes were heartbreaking: mothers and fathers sleeping in the streets and going door-to-door begging for money to pay for tests and medicines.

It was so awful that my mother organized collections with her friends and neighbors to help pay for strangers' treatments. All the doctors came to know her for her efforts, and they would send the neediest patients to our door. She would hand out cash to those who could show receipts for medical services and medications. I remember sometimes she would send me to the corner drugstore for medicines that we'd hand out together.

But there was never enough money. One day, in my innocence, I asked my mother why the government did not pay for the treatment of the poorest people. It was a question I was still asking when I became Mexico's president.

That's why, when I took office, I decided to follow the folk wisdom and establish health as the foundation of my social platform. For my government, health came first.

Talk is never enough, however. Improved access to health care is a common campaign promise, particularly for candidates in developing countries. Politicians never really elaborate on these promises, and when they take office they make no structural changes to budgetary priorities. This is where change needs to occur.

If a government leader truly wishes to make health care a priority, the only way to take this beyond good intentions is with significant economic resourcing. In Mexico we often joke that "love that is not reflected in the budget is not true love." I remember talking to my transition team and asking them what it would take to reach universal health coverage in the ensuing six years. The answer was unanimous: "It is impossible, Mr. President."

But I insisted my staff prepare budgets for the next six years starting with this goal. I ordered them to design our budget beginning with my priorities instead of making small changes to the previous year's budget. We assigned what was needed to health care first and then moved on to subsequent priorities. It's true that we made sacrifices and cuts to other programs, some of them important and others that were not very useful. But health was always the top priority.

During my first year in office we doubled the budget for Seguro Popular, a program that offers health services for people that do not have health insurance. Six years later, at the end of my time in office, the budget for Seguro Popular was five times bigger and the number of people insured under this program had grown from 16 million to 53 million.

Ultimately this investment helped raise the number of Mexicans with health insurance from 60 million to 106 million, out of a population of 112 million. We achieved universal health care, a feat no one had thought possible at Mexico's stage of economic development. To give you an idea of our impact, consider that when I took office, seven out of ten children with leukemia died; by the end of my administration, seven out of ten survived. Other health areas also improved, with total health spending rising by 105%. We hired 33,000 doctors and 48,000 nurses. We built 1,264 new clinics and hospitals and rebuilt or expanded 2,400 more.

Of course, it took more than money. We had to increase coordination between the federal government, which paid for the services, and state governments, which provided them. My government also had to increase coordination between the different public health providers, including the government workers health service, the health ministry hospitals, and the private sector insurance providers, to avoid duplication.

These challenges required leadership and personal follow-up. As a social and governmental priority, it took time and money.

Finally, through public programs, we worked hard to make sure patients learned what they were entitled to—a break from the longstanding tradition of patients owing a debt of gratitude to the government for providing assistance. Patients became the government's best allies in ensuring that local providers actually provided the services for which they were being paid.

In the end, the solution was not simple, but clear: we established health as the priority and devoted enough resources to realize the changes we wanted to see. These changes have not only strengthened our health system, but they have made a meaningful difference in people's lives and well-being. While we are far from finished with this work, my hope is that this success will inspire other governments to make universal access to health care a real priority and not just a pipe dream.

Felipe Calderón was President of Mexico from 2006 to 2012.

Chapter 18

Committing to Unbridled Collaboration

RAY CHAMBERS

Collaborative problem-solving is the only way we will achieve global health goals, but getting there requires that we rethink and rework the incentives that drive global health solutions.

One thing I've observed across my career—as a businessman, as a philanthropist, and as a UN Special Envoy—is that when we collaborate, we solve problems more creatively and meet challenges more successfully. If the global community could tackle its biggest health challenges with a spirit of unbridled collaboration, we would find ourselves living in a healthier and more equitable world.

The Millennium Development Goals (MDGs) provide a powerful example of collaborative goal-setting. In 2000, nearly all the world's countries agreed to eight ambitious goals that effectively established a global partnership to end extreme poverty. The achievements resulting from this shared road map are among the great triumphs in human history. Child and maternal mortality has declined dramatically, we have witnessed unimaginable progress in turning the tide on HIV/AIDS, and the ancient scourges of malaria and tuberculosis, though still taking far too many lives, are within sight of defeat.

The work behind us has not been easy, but the work ahead will require us to think far more expansively about ways to support collaborative problem-solving. Curing cancer; eradicating malaria, tuberculosis, and HIV/AIDS; a world free from preventable child deaths; genetic medicine tailored to every individual—each of these dreams is possible, but only if we can unlock the power of collaboration.

One critical step toward becoming more collaborative is understanding and then reworking the incentives that drive problem-solving in health. As a businessman, I recognize the importance of a competitive marketplace. But when it comes to goals serving humanity rather than the bottom line, business motivations such as profit, market leadership, and shareholder value can be much harder to achieve. Many of our most serious or intractable health challenges are found in parts of the world that are least able to pay the market rates that incentivize those developing or implementing solutions.

In competitive marketplaces, advantage is typically gained by having something others don't have: patents, top talent, hard-won relationships, available financial resources. Yet so many of our current health challenges will only be solved when those assets are shared beyond the "owner" who secured them. So we must encourage—and, ultimately, require—unfettered access to health knowledge and data developed by governments, academic institutions, private industry, and civil society. We must promote the concept that all health research and knowledge should, as much as possible, serve the common good.

There are many tested approaches to driving collaboration in health, and we should take the best learning from recent experiences and play them forward. So-called "product development partnerships" use public and philanthropic funds to incentivize research and development for health solutions that otherwise offer limited profit potential. "Patent pools" have been created—notably, in health, for HIV/AIDS—to help ensure that patented drugs are sub-licensed to generic manufacturers so they can be made more widely available where most needed and at a lower cost. Millions of lives have been saved and millions of HIV infections are being averted because collaborative agreements have enabled dramatic price reductions.

A particularly welcome tool for unlocking collaboration in health research has been the stipulation of unfettered access to data as a requirement for receiving health research funds. This should be the standard default.

In addition to unlocking the forces of research and development collaboration, we must also encourage collaboration across sectors, across silos, and across barriers that we may consider too entrenched to change. We miss opportunities and squander resources when we solve for health in isolation from education, from environment, and from human rights. People working in and leading different humanitarian sectors should regularly reach out to colleagues in different fields, especially when they share commonalities such as geography, populations, and even research facilities and funding sources.

Finally, there are public–private collaborations which have been championed in so many innovative ways in global health. The assets of the private sector—innovation, influence, access, financial acumen—can be catalytic when combined with the society-wide interests of government. With an eye on achievement of the MDGs, I was particularly impressed when I witnessed the Nigerian Ministry of Health partner with the Nigerian Private Sector Health Alliance to align their health plans and approaches in the quest to save hundreds of thousands of lives by the end of 2015. I applaud government, corporate, and philanthropic leaders who recognize the catalytic impact that can result from collaboratively building on their strengths and mitigating each sector's weaknesses.

Healthy populations are essential for robust, equitable, and stable societies. Let's commit to unlocking the forces of collaboration, wherever possible, so that all people benefit from improved health.

Ray Chambers is the UN Secretary-General's Special Envoy for Financing the Health Millenium Development Goals and for Malaria and former Chairman of Wesray Capital Corporation.

Chapter 19

A New Philanthropy

GERALD L. CHAN

A new kind of financial capital is needed for translating science into products that benefit public health.

The dawn of the twenty-first century brought with it a golden age of life science. This golden age came about as a fruit of Western governments investing generously in the scientific enterprise for over half a century.

Concomitant and building upon this golden age of life science is another golden age of translating such new science into products for the improvement of human health, products such as vaccines, diagnostics, drugs, or medical devices. Breakthroughs in science in the late twentieth century gave birth to the biotechnology industry, which was founded specifically for turning scientific discoveries into products. This mission was, and still is, both exceedingly risky and expensive—risky because human biology is complex; expensive because a rigorous regulatory regime must be in place if society is to be assured that the medical products that come to market for public consumption are up to a sufficient standard of safety and efficacy. Against huge odds, the biotechnology industry has survived and thrived.

In earlier times when the output of science was the bottleneck, pharmaceutical companies were able to provide adequate capital for commercializing such output. With the advent of the golden age of life science, the bottleneck is no longer science but the amount of capital available for downstream development. Providers of such capital now choose which projects to fund among a panoply of scientific discoveries. On what grounds are these choices made?

The nature of capital in a market economy is to maximize financial return. Pharmaceutical companies have to do this for their shareholders. The venture capitalists who serve the function of gathering capital from the private sector to support the biotech industry are under the same mandate. This mandate constrains the industry, developing only products whose markets are large even if the unit price is moderate, or products which can command extremely high pricing even if their markets are small. Products for curative medicine are more likely to fulfill either one of these two criteria, but not products that serve public health goals. Consider vaccines—undoubtedly the single class of medical products that has had the greatest impact on public health. For many years, pharmaceutical companies did not engage in developing new vaccines because the financial return from doing so was far inferior to developing novel oncology drugs, anti-inflammatory agents, or replacement enzymes for rare genetic diseases.

The tension between maximizing profit and maximizing public health impact will remain unresolved so long as the shareholders of a company have as their sole purpose the reaping of financial gain. Indeed, if that shareholder was a pension fund, its purpose cannot be otherwise. The pension fund manager's obligation is toward the pensioners, not toward the public, which needs products for better health.

The translation of life science into products serving public health goals calls for a new kind of financial capital that has the following characteristics. First, its expectation for financial return is negligible, if any. Second, its time horizon is long, commensurate with the multi-year time horizon of developing regulated medical products. Third, the risk tolerance of this capital is high as the projects it supports are technically challenging. Fourth, this capital should be run by scientists with experience in product development. Using vaccines again as an example, we have yet to succeed in developing vaccines for many prevalent infectious diseases which plague both the developed and developing world today in spite of multiple attempts with diverse approaches. It is not surprising that the efficacy requirements for vaccines must be high. As vaccines are administered to large populations of people who are not sick, oftentimes children, the safety hurdle is necessarily much higher than that which can pass for drugs administered to patients whose disease would be fatal if untreated. On top of such onerous challenges, vaccines cannot be expensive if they are to be widely adopted throughout the world.

The financial capital that possesses these characteristics may be considered as philanthropic capital. An early example of such philanthropic capital can be found in the work of certain patient advocacy groups. The Cystic Fibrosis Foundation has invested $75 million USD in collaboration with a biotech company to develop the first drug approved for cystic fibrosis. For this foundation, any expectation for financial return is strictly ancillary to developing a drug for cystic fibrosis patients.

The postindustrial new economy has produced enormously wealthy people who are younger and more activist in disposition. To satiate their desire for impact, this wealth needs to be guided into translating novel science into products with public health benefits to the world. Humanitarian aid can produce immediately visible benefits; science is the one lever that can produce large-scale, high-impact, and long-term benefits for global health.

Rather than naming hospital wings or university buildings, why not have a new vaccine named after the philanthropist who funded that vaccine's development?

Gerald L. Chan is the co-founder of Morningside Group.

Chapter 20

Climate's Big Health Warning

MARGARET CHAN

Climate change threatens health directly, but it also highlights the need for health systems that are resilient to any unpredictable change in the economy, the environment, and society.

People in most parts of the world are getting healthier and living longer. But there is no guarantee that this favorable trend will continue into the future. The widespread rise in life expectancy is driving population growth, accompanied in some places by widening inequalities in income and consumption, and by deteriorating environments. Climate change is one facet of environmental change, and the interplay between climate, the environment, and population has uncertain consequences for human health in the coming decades.

Climate change may hold some advantages for health, but most of the effects are expected to be negative. Although no single, weather-related event can be linked with certainty to climate change, the types of adverse effects we can expect have been described consistently and persuasively. Among the many negative effects, higher average temperatures will increase the frequency of extreme heat events and raise levels of air pollution, leading to more deaths from heart disease, stroke, and respiratory conditions, particularly among the growing number of elderly people. Warmer temperatures are expected to lengthen the transmission seasons and perhaps expand the geographical ranges of infectious agents carried by insect vectors, such as mosquitoes. As the temperatures of the oceans, seas, and lakes rise, the distribution of fish and the opportunities for fishing are changing in unpredictable ways.

Increasingly unpredictable rainfall patterns will affect the supply of safe, fresh water, adding to the risk of diarrheal diseases, still a major killer of young children. With more than half of the world's population residing within 60 kilometers of the sea, rising sea levels will cause floods and physical injuries, damage homes, and disrupt health services. In contrast, the world's arid regions are likely to experience further water shortages. Changes in temperature and rainfall are expected to widen the area affected by drought and increase the frequency and duration of extreme droughts. Water scarcity in turn leads to crop failures, undernutrition, and even famine.

From the perspective of health, these diverse risks have three menacing characteristics. First, climate change is most likely to exacerbate existing health hazards, especially for those people who are already most vulnerable. Second, the threats to health associated with climate change will take many forms—from a more dangerous physical environment to the worsening quality of air and water. And third, there is great uncertainty in the timing, location, and magnitude of climate's harmful effects.

Among the responses to climate change, mitigation is critical, particularly in limiting the production of greenhouse gases and fine particulate matter. Mitigation will bring many health benefits, including the reduction of air pollution indoors and outdoors. But for those who are most concerned with health, the direct challenges are in adaptation—building resilience, not only to the effects of climate but to social and environmental changes of all kinds. Climate's big health warning is one that is difficult to anticipate: today's hard-pressed health services should prepare for a greater number of unpredictable challenges in the future.

The threats highlighted by climate change call for a set of actions to safeguard health. The first is to strengthen health systems where they are weakest. This means building robust and responsive services for primary care, prevention, and for health care in emergencies. It means installing early warning and monitoring systems in the places at greatest risk, including coastal areas and desert fringes. The second imperative is to combine forces for more effective responses. The World Health Organization, the intergovernmental agency I lead, can play a big part in preparing for and responding to the effects of climate on health. But the World Health Organization works most effectively in coordination with other United Nations entities, among many other collaborators. The third course of action is to reinforce the science of climate change and our understanding of the way climate affects health. This is maximizing knowledge to minimize risk.

But even now, we already know enough about climate, environmental change, and population vulnerability to draw one firm conclusion: concerted action to build resilient systems is a sure investment in health today, and a safe bet against our uncertain future.

Margaret Chan is Director-General of the World Health Organization and former Director of Health of Hong Kong.

Chapter 21

Tackling Obesity and Overweight

HELEN CLARK

Lessons from past public health reforms can help shape our approach to food and consumption.

One of the greatest challenges to public health is the global obesity epidemic. Between 1980 and 2013, the combined prevalence of overweight and obese individuals rose by approximately 28% for adults and an alarming 47% for children. We now live in a world where 2.1 billion people—nearly one-third of the entire population—are overweight or obese.

Transnational food and beverage companies have thriving markets in both the developed and developing worlds. The consumption of foods high in fats, salts, and processed sugars contributes a great deal to premature death and disease. The public policy choices made—or not made—around the reputation of these foods are therefore very significant.

The successes and failures of tobacco control efforts over the past decade give some insight into how unhealthy foods and beverages might be tackled. The World Health Organization's Framework Convention on Tobacco Control is an important international, legally binding treaty on a health issue. It has proven to be invaluable in equipping governments with the tools they need to fundamentally alter the environments in which tobacco production, sales, and consumption are shaped.

To combat obesity, a similar package of policies on pricing, product labeling, taxation, and marketing should be explored.

Policies to tackle obesity must also respond to issues of inequality, which are common to all health and development challenges. In most countries, for example, women are more likely to be obese than are men. Obesity patterns also mirror inequality in income and education. In my home country of New Zealand, where nearly one in three adults is obese and 34% are overweight, our indigenous Maori population is hit the hardest. Nearly half of all Maori adults are now obese, and mortality in middle-age from cardiovascular disease for Maori is two to three times that for non-Maori. In the wider South Pacific, nearly 70% of adults are obese. This situation is rightly considered to be a crisis.

In the face of such challenges, it would be wrong simply to lay the blame on personal choices. Instead, we must understand that behaviors are shaped by environment, which can be improved if policies on trade, governance, consumption, and urbanization work for, and not against, public health.

Fulfilling our global commitment to halt the rise in obesity by 2025 will require the scaling-up of noncommunicable disease prevention and treatment strategies. Equally important to success will be striking a better balance between economic and public health interests.

With political will and cross-sectoral public policy reform, we could make a positive impact on our neighborhoods, supermarkets, schools, and kitchen tables. Consumers do move away from processed foods toward healthier options, such as fruits, vegetables, and lean sources of protein, when encouraged to do so. Taxes on sugar-sweetened beverages, for example, could make a significant impact. Governments can prioritize human development through public policies that promote health and address inequalities. The bleaker alternative is the maintenance of the social and economic conditions that allow obesity rates to soar.

Helen Clark is the Administrator of the United Nations Development Programme and was Prime Minister of New Zealand from 1999 to 2008.

Chapter 22

Preventing Premature Deaths

BILL CLINTON

Broad-based partnerships are crucial to reduce the burden of premature deaths and advance a healthier future in all countries.

This year, approximately 36 million people around the world will die from preventable, treatable, or reversible conditions: nearly 100,000 people a day, from children in the developing world suffering from infections related to dirty water to middle-aged residents of wealthy nations succumbing to heart disease.

The burden of disease still falls heaviest on the poor. Nearly 80% of deaths from noncommunicable diseases occur in developing countries. If we want to build a world of shared opportunities, shared responsibilities, and shared futures, we can't afford to leave anyone behind.

Virtually every premature death can be prevented through interventions that are affordable and effective. As my friend Paul Farmer said, we need to be sure that "the fruits of science serve everyone." Harnessing our collective resources and know-how to prioritize wellness and facilitate early treatment of illness is the simplest, most cost-effective thing we can do to dramatically improve health on a global scale.

Growing prosperity has increased life expectancy overall, but far too many of us are dying from an unhealthy lifestyle. Unless we are killed in an accident, conflict, or natural disaster, most of us play a hand in our own undoing. Noncommunicable diseases like cancer, and chronic conditions like heart disease, diabetes, and asthma, are the leading causes of death on every continent but Africa, where if current trends continue, by 2030, they will be the leading cause of death there too.

For countries struggling under the double burden of poverty and disease, malnutrition, contaminated drinking water, diarrhea, and poor sanitation, plus high rates of HIV/AIDS, TB, and malaria, still pose tremendous threats to survival and daunting challenges to people who need lifesaving treatments that wealthier nations take for granted.

While the challenges vary from country to country, governments, NGOs, and private business can form networks of creative cooperation everywhere to implement large-scale, game-changing strategies that lengthen lives.

For example, diarrhea kills an estimated 760,000 children under age 5 worldwide. The Clinton Health Access Initiative is working alongside the governments of Uganda and Nigeria, and with donors such as ELMA and the Norwegian Agency for Development Cooperation, to increase the uptake of oral rehydration salts and zinc. By educating mothers and health-care workers about this simple, effective treatment, we can prevent most diarrhea-related deaths for about 50 cents per child. We are also working with the IKEA and Gates foundations on similar projects in Kenya and India. Through innovative distribution channels, we've been able to reach more than 120,000 rural medical providers in India with both information and lifesaving medication.

Public–private partnerships in Rwanda and Ethiopia are reducing infant mortality and malnutrition by teaming with local farmers to produce nutritious and affordable foods that both strengthen childhood health and increase farmers' incomes, proving that prevention is not only good sense but good economics.

In countries where the biggest challenges to preventing premature death are organizational, offering access to inexpensive treatments is not enough. That's why Rwanda's Human Resources for Health program, including CHAI and several US medical schools, is building integrated systems to ensure that adequate numbers of workers are being trained, retained, and deployed to the communities in which they are most needed. As a result, Rwanda is on its way to meeting its goal of creating a high-quality, self-sustaining health-care system by 2020.

In wealthy nations, the challenge is to adapt old systems to new realities, replacing illness-based care with policies that emphasize wellness at all stages of life. For example, chronic diseases like heart disease, obesity, and type 2 diabetes are now responsible for 7 of 10 deaths and 75% of health-care spending in the United States. We're now seeing type 2 diabetes in children as young as 8 years old. Over the past two decades, the number of people suffering from diabetes has tripled, affecting more than 25 million Americans; it is now the leading cause of a number of complications, including kidney failure and blindness.

But here, too, we've found that partnerships can achieve meaningful results in improving health. My foundation and the American Heart Association founded Alliance for a Healthier Generation to combat childhood obesity. Today, we are working in over 23,500 schools with more than 14 million students. There's been a decrease of more than 90% in the total calories in drinks shipped to our schools' cafeterias and vending machines. It was just a simple agreement by people who found a way to do business and improve our kids' health.

Preventing and reversing disease is tough work that requires patience, flexibility, and the coordinated efforts of many people. Every year brings new challenges, but we have never been in a better position to develop and deploy low-cost, high-impact responses.

The best thing we can do to advance a healthier future is to prevent premature death.

Bill Clinton is former President of the United States.

Chapter 23

HIV Treatment, a Moral Duty

PAUL COLLIER

HIV is now a preventable and manageable disease; government must lead the way on both fronts.

Before the advent of antiretroviral therapies in the 1990s, being infected with HIV was equivalent to a death sentence. Now, thanks to remarkable advances in medical research, people who are HIV-positive can lead relatively normal lives as long as they take antiretroviral drugs properly. The increasing availability of effective drugs at a moderate cost has fundamentally changed the ethics of HIV treatment. The median cost of treatment in low-income countries is now as low as $792 USD a year, including personnel and laboratory costs. In turn, this new ethics has long-term economic consequences on the financial sustainability of poor countries with high-prevalence rates. I am part of a team of economists and health specialists who are currently researching these implications.

If an individual can be saved from death at around this cost, then given global incomes, it is reasonable to invoke a moral duty of rescue. Such a duty is widely accepted, even if wider responsibilities may be denied. For example, everyone will agree that there is a duty to pull a drowning child out of a pond if one has the power to do so. However, many would not accept a responsibility to build a fence around the pond to prevent the risk that a child might die because of the negligence of the parents. Unlike wider responsibilities, the duty of rescue is limited only by feasibility, not by preferences.

The reduction in the cost of treating HIV-positive people has major implications for the financing of HIV policies. First, treatment achieves containment rather than cure. HIV is a long-term viral infection that causes the progressive failure of the immune system, and for which no definitive cure yet exists. Antiretroviral therapies reduce the viral load in the blood of HIV-positive individuals, thereby allowing their immune systems to recover, thereby decreasing the likelihood of deadly opportunistic infections and cancers. However, even if antiretroviral drugs are taken properly, HIV does not fully disappear from infected blood, and viral loads rebound if treatment is stopped. Antiretroviral treatment against HIV needs to be sustained for the long run, making this more similar to the management of a long-term chronic disease than to the one-time treatment of a fatal disease. This difference has important economic implications for the long-term cost of the duty to rescue for HIV. Offering lifelong antiretroviral treatment to HIV-positive people needing treatment generates a long-term financial liability.

This begs the question, who should bear this duty to rescue? Primarily, this responsibility rests with government. Some African governments can afford to meet this duty. For example, in Botswana, the long-term cost of treating all infected citizens would be equivalent to increasing the national debt by around 27% of GDP. While this is substantial, Botswana is a lightly indebted middle-income country and can afford the liability. Once this duty to rescue has been recognized, it leads to a second implication for HIV policies—the appropriate allocation of resources to prevention. It is economically sensible to increase spending on prevention up to the point at which an extra dollar so spent reduces the future fiscal liability by a dollar. Hence, instead of prevention and treatment being viewed as competing demands on the health budget, they become complementary.

For some governments, however, the fiscal implications of the duty to rescue would increase their debt burdens beyond sustainability. For example, if the government of Malawi was to take on this same obligation, the fiscal burden would be equivalent to extra debt of over 170% of its GDP. Such a burden has already been recognized by the international community as not feasible. In this case, the duty to rescue does not evaporate, but rather shifts from Malawian taxpayers to international taxpayers through international aid. The same principle concerning expenditure on prevention and treatment now applies to aid donors: it is sensible for them to spend on prevention up to the level at which an extra dollar reduces future expenditures on treatment by a dollar.

Between countries like Botswana and those like Malawi, there is a range in which the duty to rescue should be shared between local taxpayers and international donors. In such cases, another important principle applies: however the costs of treatment are shared between the two parties, the costs of prevention should be shared in the same way. Only then can we avoid moral hazard. If domestic taxpayers were to fund prevention while donors funded treatment, there would be too little incentive to spend on prevention.

These core principles of sustainable financing and shared fiscal burdens for prevention and treatment should be at the heart of all HIV policies.

Paul Collier is Professor of Economics and Public Policy and Co-Director of the Centre for the Study of African Economies at the University of Oxford.

Chapter 24

The Power of Science

FRANCIS S. COLLINS

Strong support for scientific research translates into major benefits for human health around the globe.

Scientific research is the engine that drives health advances. If future world leaders would keep that simple concept in mind when making decisions about where and how to invest their resources, the health of humankind would improve substantially over the next 50 years and beyond.

Some may question the value of this science-centric perspective for global health. Yet I am convinced that rigorous, well-designed research is essential not only for the discovery of new ways to detect, treat, and prevent disease, but also for the most efficient development and cost-effective dissemination of such advances to the world's poorest peoples. The remarkable progress made in genomics, bioengineering, and many other scientific fields over the past decade has given rise to innovative technologies now being used to help many different populations in many different settings.

For instance, some of the technologies that spurred the molecular biology revolution are now being put to work in developing countries to diagnose diseases more swiftly and accurately. These "point-of-care" diagnostics include a DNA-amplification test that makes it possible to diagnose tuberculosis and detect drug resistance within 90 minutes. This means patients can start taking effective drugs on the same day they are tested, rather than waiting several months for traditional lab results or starting costly ineffective therapy that must be changed if their tuberculosis strain proves to be drug-resistant. If deployed globally, this test would save an estimated 15 million lives by 2050.

On the near horizon, mobile health technology is already beginning to realize its potential to improve medical care in poor and remote areas. Researchers have developed a quarter-sized, lens-less microscope that, when connected to a mobile phone, can beam high-quality images of cells and microbes halfway around the globe to computers that can automatically interpret the images. An even more affordable option is a paper microscope that costs about 50 cents to produce and requires no power supply. Bioengineers designed this "use and throw away" device, which uses a spherical glass micro-lens to magnify samples up to 2,000-fold, specifically to address the challenge of quickly and accurately diagnosing malaria and other parasitic diseases in low-resource settings.

Science-based technology is also critical to disease prevention. Vaccines have made possible some of our greatest advances in global health, but we must keep scientific knowledge moving forward if we are to create the next generation of vaccines—vaccines capable of preventing HIV infection, malaria, and other equally formidable foes. For example, thanks to basic research that expanded understanding of the influenza virus, I am confident that a "universal flu vaccine" will be developed in the next decade that will provide long-term protection against multiple flu strains, effectively disarming the threat of future worldwide flu epidemics.

While infectious diseases remain a significant problem, low-income countries face many other serious health challenges. In fact, cancer, heart disease, diabetes, and other noncommunicable diseases are now among the fastest growing causes of death and disability in the developing world. It will take creative research to identify and implement the right tools to tackle this daunting—and potentially very costly—array of diseases in resource-poor countries. High on this agenda must be research to develop and test interventions that will significantly reduce smoking rates.

To succeed, we will need the most forward-thinking minds in all parts of the world to work together in highly innovative ways. One such endeavor is the Human Heredity and Health in Africa (H3Africa) initiative, in which the US National Institutes of Health and the Wellcome Trust are supporting population-based studies in Africa of common chronic disorders as well as infectious diseases. H3Africa is enabling African researchers to take advantage of new approaches to understand genetic and nongenetic factors that contribute to risk of illness. Not only will this project help Africans, but, because Africa is the cradle of humanity, what is learned about genetic variation and disease on that continent will have an impact on the health of populations around the globe.

Indeed, scientific knowledge does not travel only from developed countries to low-income countries—it is a two-way street from which the entire world stands to benefit. Recently, some of the most innovative and cost-effective advances have arisen from research reflecting the needs and ideas of people in poorer countries. From India alone have come high-performance prosthetic knee joints for amputees that cost only $20, lower-cost intraocular lenses for cataract surgery, and handheld devices that have cut the cost of electrocardiograms to $1.

As encouraging as these early successes may be, we cannot afford complacency. Much remains to be done if we want people in every corner of the world to be enjoying longer, healthier lives 50 years from now. We need far more young creative minds—be they in Boston or Botswana, Beijing or Bangladesh—to tap into the power of science to explore questions of vital importance to human health. Together, the energy and vision of a robust global scientific community can make a profound difference in one of humanity's noblest goals: improving the health of all the world's peoples.

Francis S. Collins is Director of the US National Institutes of Health and former head of the Human Genome Project.

Chapter 25

Whose Life Is It?

NIGEL CRISP

To treat today's global disease burden effectively, we must shift to health systems and health care that engage and empower the patient.

Whose life is it anyway? Whose health? Whose decisions? As a friend of mine observed, "When did we decide to outsource our health to the professionals?"

For centuries people relied for their health and health care on the wisdom of their community and the care of their families, churches, and charities. There was little help available from health professionals, whose skills were uncertain and whose knowledge was patchy at best. Now, with medical science and the professions having advanced so spectacularly, the positions are reversed. Mighty medicine and powerful health systems dominate our lives in the West to the extent that many professionals now talk about the necessity to engage and empower patients. Three recent developments show that this need is becoming ever more important.

Firstly, the main causes of death globally are now long-term chronic conditions, such as respiratory and heart disease, diabetes, and cancers. Even 50 years ago most deaths were caused by infections and trauma and many children died in the first five years of life. Now, these chronic diseases are becoming major problems even in low- and middle-income countries—as they become more affluent and their lifestyles change accordingly. Unlike infectious diseases which could be treated with vaccines or several courses of treatment, today's surge in noncommunicable diseases require significant lifestyle changes by patients. As such, it is important now more than ever before that patients are actively involved in designing their treatment plans, including nutrition and exercise.

Secondly, the World Health Organization's Commission on the Social Determinants of Health demonstrated that the way society is organized impacts health. It revealed how individuals' chances of healthy lives were affected by education, family life, housing, employment, income and social status, as well as access to medicines and health services. These differences are seen between countries but also within countries as, for example, a recent study showed that black Bostonians live on average 6.6 years less (for men) and 4.9 years (for women) less than white ones. Moreover, it is now clear that the stress of living every day with pressures from the need to find food or work—as well as from discrimination and powerlessness—have direct physiological effects on the body. As such, providing patient-centered care involves not only considering patients' physiological symptoms but recognizing that much of a person's health depends on factors beyond the professionals' direct control.

Thirdly, patients' engagement in their own care has direct and measurable benefits for their health and well-being. A recent analysis of 132 reviews published in the *British Medical Journal*, for example, cited cases of improvements in quality and cost of care with evidence of improved adherence to treatment, better outcomes, and greater satisfaction.

These insights are leading to a slow burning revolution in health promotion and health care as citizens around the world start to take initiative and change the system. Many examples come from low- and middle-income countries where people without the resources—and crucially, the baggage and vested interests—of the West are using community assets to tackle health problems. Mothers2Mothers in southern Africa engages women with HIV to help pregnant women with the virus ensure that they don't pass it on to their children. BRAC in Bangladesh mobilized rural women in a campaign to ensure that rehydration therapy was available to all children in the country—with inspiring results.

Extraordinary innovations are also happening in wealthier countries with hospitals like Massachusetts General and the Mayo Clinic developing patient-aids that guide clinicians and patients together through decision-making. England is introducing patient-controlled budgets for people with chronic diseases and long-term disabilities so that they can make the crucial choices about what matters to them. In Sweden some patients now do their own dialysis in hospital units. In Holland, ParkinsonNet engages patients alongside doctors in care and decision-making. Meanwhile, patients themselves have set up their own information exchanges, helping each other learn about new treatments and engage in self-care, self-monitoring, and self-diagnosis enabled by technology.

I believe that the next revolution in health and well-being will come about when these sorts of initiatives take center stage. They will precipitate a much-needed change in services and professional education, both of which were designed for the problems of the last century.

Only through accelerating and supporting these patient-driven and patient-centered developments can we expect to see any real slow down of the growing epidemic of noncommunicable diseases and improvement in health for all people worldwide.

Nigel Crisp is a member of the UK House of Lords and former permanent secretary of the UK Department of Health and chief executive of the English National Health Service.

Chapter 26

Security for Our Shared Home

SURAYA DALIL

Conflict and insecurity pose lasting negative consequences for human health and development and should be addressed both nationally and globally.

I was in my fourth-grade classroom on a spring day in April when the first shootings and air strikes started in Kabul. Little did I understand then that it was the start of a political revolution that would shake the entire country and lead to years of conflict.

This conflict has changed the lives of millions of Afghans living in an already economically poor country. We have experienced chronic suffering, displacement, physical disability, trauma, and been driven to exile and death. My country has suffered decades of lost development. Many Afghans believe that geography and geopolitics caused the Afghan crisis, but whatever the cause, the conflict has had regional and global impact.

Looking at that prolonged conflict and current international events, my fellow Afghans and I have become increasingly aware of the importance of security for the nation's development and its impact on health. Insecurity affects human resources, infrastructure, behavior, morality, economy, governance, and accountability—all of which, in turn, affect health. While insecurity causes trauma and reduces access to health care, its long-term impacts are much more severe. These include mental health issues, lost generations, poor rule of law, and lack of faith in government, all of which breed more insecurity and perpetuate a vicious cycle.

Addressing poverty is the first imperative in improving human security and, by extension, health outcomes. Poverty, deprivation, and social injustice have manifested in the form of social unrest and conflict in parts of Afghanistan. In countries plagued by war and insecurity, young generations with little education and no employment opportunities are a soft target for recruitment by extreme religious groups. Some religious schools and madrassas have progressively become homes for children from poor families, by enrolling students for free board and education. In many of those schools violence and combat are taught rigorously and students graduate to become insurgents.

Secondly, effective governance is fundamental in ensuring accountability and improving safety and security. The government's role in addressing basic human needs, reducing social inequalities, protecting citizens' rights (especially the rights of women and children), and providing socioeconomic development opportunities is at the core of building public trust and national development. The government's policies toward creating an enabling environment for civil society as a voice for change are important in the overall leadership function and improving social trust.

Although economic growth, equality, and governance are country-specific realities, the long-term impact of insecurity is widespread. In today's world, security has a global dimension. Conflict and violence, as well as peace and development, reinforce each other and extend beyond the confines of national borders. Improving security for better health involves concerted national action that is supported and mirrored at the global level. These actions include promoting a deeper understanding of different faiths—both between and within religions—recognizing diversity, creating opportunities for growth, developing a shared interest for human and global security, and enhancing international harmony and coherence.

We all have made remarkable progress in the last half century in technology, telecommunication, air travel, and accessing outer space. The time has now come to make a commitment for peace and prosperity in the world that is our shared home.

Suraya Dalil is a former Minister of Public Health of Afghanistan.

Chapter 27

The Drugs Don't Work

SALLY C. DAVIES

Modern medicine is under threat as bacteria develop resistance to antibiotics and the pipeline of new drugs is empty.

Antibiotics underpin all of modern medicine, from curing common sore throats to facilitating transplants, cancer care, and major surgery. Yet bacteria continue to develop resistance to these essential drugs, and their resistant clones proliferate by natural selection and by their ability to pass resistant genes between themselves. Meanwhile, many patients in low- and middle-income countries with treatable infections have no access to effective antibiotics.

While resistance is a natural phenomenon, certain societal behaviors foster its development. These include the use of antibiotics for nonbacterial infections, using the wrong antibiotic, taking the wrong dose, stopping treatment prematurely, and/or using one antibiotic alone rather than several in combination. The current pattern of resistance has been likened to an arms race between humans and bacteria, and it is crucial that we stay ahead of the enemy.

Antimicrobial resistance is a global problem affecting every country. Today globalization and increased air travel allow new resistant strains to cross the world in a matter of days. For example, the New Delhi Metallo-beta-lactamase-1 (NDM-1) strain spread in 2008 from India to 17 countries within a year. Increasing numbers of multidrug-resistant and extensively drug-resistant forms of tuberculosis are also reason for concern. A recent World Health Organization report acknowledges the very high rates of resistant bacteria causing common infections in all regions. Bacteria that we had once vanquished are making a powerful comeback.

While limiting human antibiotic use to necessary and appropriate circumstances reduces resistance, the reality is that over 70% of antibiotics sold worldwide are used in animals. This highlights another facet of this growing problem: too often, antibiotics in animals are used not to treat infection, but rather for growth promotion and as a substitute for good hygiene. Antimicrobial resistance can be passed through the food chain and from animals to humans meaning that we need rules for limiting the use of antibiotics in animals, fish farming, and agriculture.

In moving toward a solution, we must first promote proper sanitation. We must refocus both our health systems and food chains on cleaner water sources and improved hygiene practices like frequent and thorough hand-washing. These measures will reduce the incidence of infections and in turn our need for antibiotics.

Second, we must conserve existing antibiotics through stewardship programs that achieve better clinical outcomes with reduced antibiotic use. The right antibiotic should be used at the right dose for the right duration and, if appropriate, in the right combination. To ensure that this happens, antibiotics (and their precursors) should not be available over-the-counter or over-the-web, but only on prescription from a health professional who follows guidance informed by local laboratory surveillance programs. If antibiotics are to be recognized once again as lifesaving drugs, stewardship programs must take the lead in developing and enforcing stricter prescription practices.

Advancements in the fight against antimicrobial resistance are dependent on the public's awareness of the harms and consequences of antibiotics abuse and misuse. As patients, we all need to accept our doctor's professional judgment when told our illness or our child's high temperature is unlikely to be of bacterial origin—and as such unresponsive to antibiotics.

We have escaped the dire consequences of resistance until now thanks to the discovery of several key classes of antibiotics during the last century. However, over the last 25 years, the antibiotic pipeline has been running dry. Cautious estimates of the attributable deaths to antimicrobial resistance run at 25,000 per year in Europe and 23,000 per year in the United States. Today, we are in desperate need of new classes of antibiotics, innovative approaches to treat infection, and rapid affordable diagnostics to distinguish bacterial diseases from other infections. Yet there has been little investment in new antibiotics, particularly from big pharmaceutical companies, because of high research costs and relatively low reimbursement rates. Such discrepancies can only be addressed through partnerships between private and public institutions, government and nongovernmental organizations, and academia and industry. Ultimately, we need a new approach to sustain the discovery and development of antibiotics, for today and centuries to come.

As the threat of antimicrobial resistance grows, global organizations are starting to rise to the challenge. The World Health Organization, in collaboration with the Food and Agriculture Organization and the World Organization for Animal Health, is developing a strategic action plan to combat antimicrobial resistance, while also supporting countries in developing national strategies.

In spreading awareness about antimicrobial resistance, we can make it a priority on national and international political agendas and ensure that our governments are active in global efforts to curb resistance. Scientific advances over the past century have provided us with the incredible benefits of modern medicine we enjoy today, and concerted global action is the only way to protect these advances for present and future generations.

Sally C. Davies is the Chief Medical Officer of the United Kingdom.

Chapter 28

Vision 2020—and Beyond

MARK DYBUL

Global health needs a clear, bold vision for the future.

Our vision today is shaped by our past when it should be shaped by our future.

To begin, we must look at the world a decade into the future and consider the implications for global health. New geopolitical and economic powers, including Brazil, China, India, Indonesia, Mexico, South Africa, South Korea, and Turkey, will be joined by Chile, Nigeria, Vietnam, and many others to irrevocably alter the center of gravity in global affairs. In the new world, official development assistance (ODA)—the commitment of tax dollars from wealthy countries to low- and middle-income countries that has fueled global health gains—will likely end. The word "assistance" already rings hollow. It is a remnant of a paternalistic past, not of present-day partnerships, and it has no relevance for the future. Beyond the language, the foundations of ODA are on shaky ground.

High-income countries that have poured money into ODA to support the world's poorest countries will be challenged by significant shifts. Seventy percent of people living in poverty now reside in middle-income countries, compared with 24% in 1990. Many infectious and chronic diseases are now in those higher economic strata. Two-thirds of HIV and three-quarters of tuberculosis infections are already there and that trend will continue.

Part of the new vision could be a refined classification of a country's economic progress rather than the current blunt instrument of gross national income (GNI). Currently, on the path to transition from ODA, low-income countries become middle-income when their per capita GNI exceeds $1,035 USD—even by one dollar. At least for health, statistics such as the percent of people living in poverty and those with access to essential health commodities could be useful. This might allow high-income countries to accompany middle-income countries along a smooth transition to self-sufficiency.

Another challenge is the need for increased domestic spending on health. These increases are necessary to address urgent health needs, but also to maintain investments by high-income countries. Leaders in middle- and even low-income countries need the vision to see this reality and invest accordingly.

The role of the new geopolitical and emergent powers needs to be defined. They do not seem interested in following the path of ODA, perhaps because not long ago many were treated as "recipients of aid" by paternalistic development systems when, in fact, they had pioneered innovative approaches to provide health to their people. But what their new vision will be remains to be seen.

At a more granular level, individual diseases are still viewed in isolation, rather than as a part of a person's overall health. While all resources need not be bundled in one funding stream, we do need a more coordinated way of providing support to countries as they implement their national strategies. Despite significant progress, the current ODA systems and organizations are not positioned to support a broader vision for coherent health delivery. Until global health is better aligned within health-care provision, it is difficult to see how we can expand our peripheral vision to encompass key areas beyond formal health care that nonetheless have significant impact on health outcomes. These areas include cultural, legal, and structural issues, such as the fundamental inequity of young girls and women and their vulnerability to sexual violence and abuse, as well as discrimination against the LGBT community, sex workers, people who inject drugs, migratory populations, prisoners, and other marginalized groups, which fuels the HIV/AIDS pandemic. Equal access to opportunity for women as economies grow will depend on the health and education of girls. We need a new, more integrated, and inclusive vision of the peripheral boundaries of global health.

At the most granular level, our vision also seems stuck in the past. Specific prevention, care, and treatment targets are still needed to ensure success in the fight against diseases like HIV/AIDS, tuberculosis, and malaria. Recent advances in science and epidemiologic understanding, and the lessons and foundations of past investments, make transformational differences and bring epidemics under control—to convert pandemics to low-level endemicity and to end them as public health threats. Within individual disease programs, we need a new, bold vision rather than being limited by strategies developed a decade ago before significant scientific advances.

Global health's biggest challenge is a lack of vision and the audacity to look to the future, to what the world will look like, and to what that means for equitable opportunity, health, and well-being. To leave no one behind and move forward sustainably, we must reassess today's reality and plan for a future that is reflective of the world's changing social, economic, and cultural landscapes.

We did it before. We can and must do it again.

Mark Dybul is Executive Director of the Global Fund to Fight AIDS, Tuberculosis and Malaria and former US Global AIDS Coordinator responsible for overseeing the US President's Emergency Plan for AIDS Relief.

Chapter 29

Achieving Social Equity

CARISSA F. ETIENNE

To ensure better health, we must address the social determinants that impede it.

Social equity is the one thing most needed in the world for achieving better health. Evidence of pervasive and deep social, economic, and environmental inequities is ubiquitous. This perpetuates a world of unjust, unfair differences in opportunities for citizens to fulfill a dignified, rewarding, and healthy life. There is ample recognition that this broad social inequity is a structural threat to human development, sustainability, democracy, good governance, and economic growth. The adoption of an approach to health that looks at these social determinants is, indisputably, the foremost transformative insight in contemporary public health thinking, but the world has yet to see it consistently translated into policymaking. Now more than ever before, we need to launch a concerted effort to explicitly eliminate these inequities to achieve global social equity.

This fundamental change toward achieving social equity requires moving away from practicing an individual-based, behavior-centered, "risk factor" public health, and toward a broader public policy and multidisciplinary approach. Such an approach would address the interdependence of individuals and their connection with the biological, physical, social, and historical contexts in which they are born, grow, work, live, and age.

From the pioneering Lalonde Report to the works of the World Health Organization's Commission on the Social Determinants of Health, it has been widely recognized that health systems and services are, by themselves, core determinants of health. The ways in which these core societal resources are organized to fulfill public health demands may determine the level of both population health and health inequities. Universal health coverage is a feasible way for addressing these determinants and exerting the health sector's stewardship role in achieving social equity.

Worldwide, and particularly within the region of the Americas, evidence is mounting on a number of successfully implemented, country-championed, national experiences on social protection mechanisms and social inclusion policies. These include cash transfers and interventions to promote equity through health systems, where universal health coverage is a central, strategic component to which countries have committed, as reflected in World Health Assembly debates. They are powerful examples of effective responses for reducing social inequities, as well as advancing the right to health. Scaling-up these successful experiences is a concrete requirement for achieving social equity. This necessary change may demand other changes to be put in place, mainly political in nature, from advancing fairness and social justice to refocusing global health partnerships. Achieving social equity then will not only be the single most-needed *goal* in the world for achieving better health, but it will also be the rational way of practicing public health: a collective mission of assuring the conditions for people to be healthy.

Carissa F. Etienne is Director of the Pan American Health Organization.

Chapter 30

Health-Care Financing and Social Justice

PAUL FARMER

We must embrace equity as the only acceptable goal of global health delivery efforts.

After 30 years of working with thousands of colleagues around the world to advance the health of people living in poverty, it's hard to identify the one *most* impermeable barrier or one *most* promising development now before us. I should also specify that the "us" in question here includes not only Partners In Health, the organization I co-founded, but also the vast and growing numbers of people engaged in care delivery; in elaborating pro-poor policies; in building private and (especially) public capacity to address health disparities; in teaching and conducting research about these and related matters; and in mobilizing the resources necessary to knock down barriers and make promising developments available to those who might most benefit from them.

The "us" also includes those afflicted by poverty and disease, since we have much to learn from them. In many ways, we (the us in question) have an "embarrassment of riches" and need to share them equitably: hence our preference, in describing such work, for the term *global health equity,* rather than "global health" or "international health" or even "public health." Global health equity should loom large in any discussion about the world's future in 2015 and beyond, in part because it leads us to a burden-and-gap analysis: what's the burden of disease for the poorest, and what is being neglected (mind the gap!) by those who consider themselves responsible for the health and well-being of the bottom billion, or even two billion?

So what's the greatest challenge in global health equity that most people don't know about? I think it's the rather mundane-sounding topic of health-care financing and social protection. Catastrophic health expenditures—unexpected, significant health costs that can push households or entire populations into poverty—are the leading cause of destitution in much of the world and stand as the ranking challenges now before us. The barriers we face in financing health care and building safety nets, more than addressing some unknown or newly virulent or curable epidemic, are not tasks widely seen by clinicians, activists, and scientists as the chief threats to and promises of global health equity.

Given its vital importance, you'd think we might have come up with something a bit more gripping than the dull-sounding terms "health-care financing" and "social protection." There will also be those who bitterly protest that we who deliver care, or concern ourselves with the "staff, stuff, space, and systems" to do so effectively, are precisely the ones who don't know much about these issues.

But others claim they *do* know all about them. My own experience with self-proclaimed experts in health-care financing and social protection suggests that they often need some sort of vaccine to protect themselves from the chief threats to the global health equity agenda in settings of poverty. These include a failure of imagination; an unwillingness to interrogate how both *cost* and *effectiveness* are socially constructed, and how these two nouns, linked in a term—cost-effectiveness—serve all too often to shut down discussions about how best to finance the global health equity agenda. What's more, the arcane language of economics and its confident claims of causality have too often served an obfuscatory and even intimidating purpose: "Thou shalt not presume to understand health-care financing or how we should weave and hang safety nets. We have limited resources, and we will decide how best to deploy them to save the most lives."

I'll close with a concrete (in every sense) example. In January 2010, an earthquake damaged or destroyed almost all of Haiti's government facilities. The five-story Ministry of Health building was pancaked into a pile of rubble no more than one story tall, and many of Haiti's public health authorities lost their lives. Haiti's chief nursing school also collapsed, with similar or worse loss of life, as very few students or faculty survived. But how do we build back "staff, stuff, space, and systems"? Not simply by importing them (although such international solidarity is important—as are continued innovations to develop new preventives, diagnostics, and therapeutics). We rebuild by believing that safety nets are important and worth fighting for, and by linking knowledge of health-care financing to global health equity.

So why do I identify these issues as the biggest and least-known challenge before us? Because almost none of the thousands of physicians and nurses I've trained feel confident enough to interrogate the "business plans" that deem care for those without ready access to care "cost-ineffective" and "unsustainable." What is unsustainable is a model of health-care financing and safety nets that doesn't elevate global health equity as the only acceptable goal.

Paul Farmer is Co-Founder of Partners In Health, Kolokotrones University Professor at Harvard University, Chief of the Division of Global Health Equity at Brigham and Women's Hospital in Boston, and the UN Secretary-General's Special Advisor on Community-Based Medicine and Lessons from Haiti.

Chapter 31

A Global CDC and FDA

RICHARD FEACHEM

The world needs a global Center for Disease Control and a global Food and Drug Administration to deal effectively with pandemics, drug resistance, licensing, and counterfeit medicines.

It is a useful thought experiment to consider the question, "If there were a government of the world, what would it do?" The simple answer is that it would focus on the financing and provision of global public goods and the elimination or attenuation of global public bads. Global public goods and bads are issues that cannot be resolved by individual countries, but which require shared commitment, collective financing, and concerted action among most or all countries. In a globalized world, divided into numerous sovereign states, the provision of global public goods and the alleviation of global public bads has proved challenging.

At the top of the list of priorities for our imaginary world government would be global law and order, climate change, and nuclear de-proliferation. Following closely behind these priorities would come, I suggest, doing what the Centers for Disease Control and Prevention (CDC) and the Food and Drug Administration (FDA) do for the United States. I think we should create a global CDC and a global FDA.

The argument for a global CDC is self-evident and particularly relates to the emerging threats of new and modified infectious diseases. We face constant stories about SARS, Ebola, MERS (Middle Eastern Respiratory Syndrome), multiple drug-resistant bacteria (superbugs), and other scary things, mainly of viral or bacterial origin. As recent history has shown, we are not equipped to identify, contain, or cope with these new threats. The biggest threat of all, for which we are hopelessly ill-prepared and on which we spend tiny amounts of money, is pandemic flu.

A day will come when a new flu virus (H?N?) emerges, which combines the two properties that we fear most: easy human-to-human transmission and high fatality rate. It may be tomorrow, it may be in 10 years, but when pandemic flu inevitably reoccurs, the results will be utterly devastating. The current international apparatus to prevent and respond to this occurrence is woefully inadequate. A global CDC would be charged with the action necessary to avoid or attenuate this and other potential pandemics. At the same time, this international agency could take on additional global health responsibilities, including development and enforcement of treaties to limit international trade and advertising of harmful substances, such as tobacco and sugar.

The need for a global FDA is perhaps less obvious. There currently exists a nightmare journey for any developer of a new drug, vaccine, or medical device to obtain the licenses needed to market their products across the more than 200 individual countries. Country-level registration, licensing, and regulation is an extraordinarily wasteful and time-consuming process. It delays access to lifesaving medicines and technologies by many years. Some countries even demand that companies conduct local randomized controlled trials in their country to demonstrate that the medicine or device works on "their people." While in rare cases there may be genetic or other reasons to do this, most of the time it's just wasteful and unnecessary.

A global FDA would provide a one-stop shop for the worldwide licensing of new medicines, vaccines, and medical technologies. It would also aggressively address, on a global scale, the rising tsunami of counterfeit drug production and trade. Despite many conferences and international deliberations, such trade is becoming more and more common and poses a greater and greater threat to individual patients and entire populations.

Likewise, a global FDA could take strenuous action on behalf of humankind to limit the inappropriate use of antibiotics and curb the rising tide of antibiotic resistance. Prime Minister David Cameron has recently warned that this problem could take modern medicine "back to the dark ages."

So, do I hope to see a global CDC or a global FDA in my lifetime? Yes. Do I expect to see it? No. I fear that mistrust among countries, cultures, and religions is on the rise and that the unity of purpose and action needed to create such institutions will prove illusive. Regardless, we must work toward that goal and try to find a reasonable surrogate. Perhaps it would be a greatly strengthened and reorganized World Health Organization, or something else entirely. Without this change, I do expect that in my lifetime there will be a flu pandemic which will spread to 100 countries in less than 10 weeks; which will kill over 200 million people; and which will set back the global economy by trillions of dollars. Avoiding this apocalyptic scenario is surely in the interest of all people in all countries. Let us act now!

Richard Feachem is Director of the Global Health Group at the University of California, San Francisco, and was founding Executive Director of the Global Fund to Fight AIDS, Tuberculosis, and Malaria.

Chapter 32

A Universal Flu Vaccine

HARVEY V. FINEBERG

World health would benefit enormously from a universal influenza vaccine that is effective against a variety of flu strains and confers long-lasting immunity.

In a typical year, influenza causes severe illness in 5 million persons and kills about 500,000 worldwide. From time to time, perhaps three times a century on average, newly emergent strains of virus cause global pandemics in which many more are at risk. The great influenza pandemic of 1918–1919 is estimated to have taken as many as 100 million lives. The most recent pandemic, the H1N1 strain in 2009, caused only a typical number of deaths, but tended to be more severe among younger persons and thus produced a disproportionately greater loss in years of life.

The principal means of preventing annual and pandemic influenza is immunization. However, today's vaccines have many limitations.

First, because the surface antigens (markers present on the outside of viruses) that are targeted by current vaccines are variable, the formulation of vaccines must be reassessed each year based on the predominant circulating variants, and the vaccine must be administered anew every flu season.

Second, current vaccines are only about 60%–70% effective in preventing influenza and even less effective in the elderly who often are especially vulnerable to flu.

Third, the time required to produce influenza vaccines means that early outbreaks in a given year will occur before vaccines have become available.

And finally, annual global production capacity falls far short of what is needed to protect everyone in the year that a new pandemic strikes.

A superior vaccine would target conserved antigens that are part of every influenza virus. At least one such vaccine is currently undergoing early trials. A universal influenza vaccine would remain effective against a variety of flu strains and would not need to be reformulated in response to changes in the variable surface proteins of the virus. If the vaccine conferred long-lasting immunity, was highly effective in all age groups, affordable, and free of major side effects, this would transform the global preventive strategy against influenza. The annual frenzy of viral surveillance, vaccine strain selection, vaccine production, and crash immunization campaigns would be replaced by a systematic, worldwide immunization program that would provide everyone with long-term protection against the threat of influenza.

Harvey V. Fineberg is President of the Gordon and Betty Moore Foundation and former President of the Institute of Medicine, Dean of the Harvard School of Public Health, and Provost of Harvard University.

Chapter 33

Accountability Is One Big Idea

COLLEEN M. FLOOD

Monitoring and measuring health care's effectiveness will go a long way toward improving it.

Accountability is the key concept for health improvement at the global level.

What, you say? Such a dry and generic observation! Such legalese! It is true that the concept of accountability is frequently hijacked by many; hollowed out to be a meaningless, bean-counting tidbit. Sadly, great ideas are frequently so hijacked.

Nevertheless, lack of accountability is why health-care systems in the developed world are failing, and why we are so miserly with the support we think we can offer to assist the developing world. Our systems are failing because we spend enormous amounts of money for very marginal returns to health and very marginal returns to a sense of comfort and caring for those who are ill or dying. We could do infinitely more with the resources that we invest in our public and private health-care systems. The problem is at heart a problem of democracy. While we can vote our governments in and out of office from time to time, this alone is wholly insufficient to ensure that the layers of accountability we need are woven throughout our health systems. Think about what could be achieved, for example, if drug companies were held accountable and rewarded for the health they deliver as opposed to the hype. As Bill Gates writes, "You can achieve incredible progress if you set a clear goal and find a measure that will drive progress toward that goal." Such progress cannot find initial traction, however, unless and until decision-makers governing our health systems are held accountable for realizing our collective goals.

As health systems fail to deliver accountability in their internal governance structures, citizens are increasingly turning to the courts to serve this function. Legal systems around the world are taking up this task with growing enthusiasm, delivering accountability on a very selective basis. Legal scholars studying this trend have found its impact to be bafflingly erratic and unpredictable—delivering progressive results in some countries and regressive results in others. While there are differing opinions as to whether judicial review should be an option of last resort for achieving accountability in health systems, nobody to my knowledge defends courts as an option of *first* resort. They're just too messy, too costly, too unfair, and too generalized a forum to do the job that needs to be done.

The enduring concept of accountability pales in its sex appeal next to flavor-of-the-week ideas like "big data." But we already have an awful lot of data about what works and doesn't work that we don't act upon. The challenge is to galvanize all the powerful people that make up our health systems to *act* upon the data, to make the changes that we need.

There is no magic bullet as to how to weave the steel wire of accountability throughout health systems and across the public and private divide. It is a task that requires continual evolution and creative thinking in institutional design to respond to changing technologies, providers, cultures, and need. It requires an understanding that measurement is a continually evolving process and that there may be very important dimensions of health systems that are as yet difficult to measure. Achieving accountability will always and ever be a work in progress, but one that we must relentlessly strive toward.

Colleen M. Flood is a Professor of Law at the University of Ottawa and was the Scientific Director of the Canadian Institutes of Health Research's Institute of Health Services and Policy Research.

Chapter 34

The Power of Knowledge

JULIO FRENK

Scientifically derived evidence is the most powerful force to guide policies for the enlightened improvement of health systems.

Knowledge is the most powerful force for enlightened social transformation. But what shapes the ideas of power, that is to say, the assumptions, concepts, and values of those with the power to make decisions? It would be naive to assume that decision-makers are always rational in the sense of basing their conclusions strictly on objective evidence about the best means to achieve the desired ends. Often, such evidence is not available. Even when it is, the decision-maker, particularly in the public sector, must balance the weight of evidence against the economic and political feasibility of following the desired course of action.

While it is clear that decisions are made on the basis of many other forces apart from scientific information, it is also true that good evidence can steer those who have the power to decide into a better course of action. In other words, the *power of ideas* can help to shape the *ideas of power.* At the very least, sound research enhances the accountability of decision-makers, who have to consider the costs of ignoring the available data. Absent such data, the decision-maker may not even be aware of the shortcomings of his or her policies. But good evidence should not be seen mainly as a limit to the decision-maker. It can also be an empowering tool. Armed with the results of research, the decision-maker can better counter the vested interests that oppose an enlightened decision. He or she may then be more willing to assume the risks of innovation.

The value of sound research to enlightened decision-making is underscored by the wave of health system reforms that is sweeping the world. Countries at all levels of economic development and with all types of political structures are planning, implementing, or evaluating reforms in the health arena. A worldwide search for better ways of financing and delivering health care is underway. Together with economic, political, and ethical reasons, this search has been fueled by the need to find answers to the complexities posed by the epidemiologic transition, whereby many nations are facing the simultaneous burdens of old, unresolved problems and new, emerging challenges. In a context marked by change and complexity, societies are discovering that the existing formulas may no longer provide the required responses. All over the world there is a shared sense of impending innovation, as we witness what could prove to be the birth of a new paradigm for health systems.

The process of rethinking and renewing health systems needs to be illuminated by research. Most of the health gains since the twentieth century were achieved because of advances in knowledge generated by research. When translated into evidence, knowledge provides a scientific foundation for behavior modification on the part of people, for quality improvement on the part of providers, and for enlightened decisions on the part of policymakers.

There are still so many unknowns about the determinants of health system performance that a research agenda must be an integral part of every reform initiative. Every reform initiative should be seen as an experiment, the effects of which must be documented for the benefit of every other initiative, both present and future. The opportunities for reform are so few that failing to learn from them condemns us to rediscover at great cost what is already known or to repeat past mistakes. To *reform,* it is necessary to *inform,* or else one is likely to *deform.*

The only way to make learning systematic and cumulative is to build evidence into every phase of the reform process. Evidence comes into play since the formulation of a precise diagnosis that may justify the reform effort. It also helps in the development of the tools for implementing the proposed changes. Finally, research is crucial to monitor unforeseen obstacles and to evaluate the effects of reform, thus opening a new cycle of improvement.

The opportunities for evidence to play a constructive role in health system reform have been greatly enhanced by the development of new tools to gather and analyze information, which give firmer quantitative and qualitative bases for the formulation and comparison of reform options. While much progress has been made, there is still a long way to go in order to standardize and refine analytical approaches. Hence, methodological development should be granted increasing attention in the years to come.

By its very nature, this type of effort requires a global scope, since knowledge derived from research is the quintessential global public good. While every reform experience will have features that are specific to its national circumstance, there are always important lessons for other countries. Hence, there is need for concerted actions among countries in order to compare options and evaluate experiences. National initiatives will have a higher likelihood of success if they can all benefit from a global process of shared learning.

Reform and research should walk together in the quest for better health. When we can achieve this convergence, we will have at last integrated ideas and power.

Julio Frenk is Dean of the Harvard T.H. Chan School of Public Health, T & G Angelopoulos Professor of Public Health and International Development at Harvard University, and former Minister of Health of Mexico.

Chapter 35

Better Information Will Save Lives

THOMAS R. FRIEDEN

Better information about health status is essential to identify health problems and effectively target, evaluate, improve, defend, and scale up health programs.

The single most important force to improve health in our lifetime will be better access to information.

Equipped with better information, people tend to make smarter health choices, which in turn contributes to improved health outcomes. Facilitating free and open access to accurate and unbiased information is a fundamental duty of government, one that will become increasingly important as the number of sources and amount of information continue to expand.

There are at least two crucial types of health information, those rooted in epidemiology and others surrounding program management. We can make enormous progress in both of these areas. We currently lack real-time, relevant information about the most important health risks of our day. Our epidemiologic systems often report data that are delayed, incomplete, and inaccurate. Records of births and deaths cover less than half of the world's people, and nearly a billion people alive today will die without ever having a legal record of their existence. Accurate information on causes of death, what we would consider the most basic information, is even less available and reliable. As such, many of the data points used for planning and program evaluation in global health are, at best, educated guesses.

Information from public health programs is the lifeblood of monitoring, but its real-time use in public health practice is rare. Good policy decisions should be based on data. Accurate, unbiased, and relevant information generated by public health agencies is at the heart of this process. What are the biggest health needs? What interventions are possible given the resources available? Who will benefit from these interventions? How much effort is needed to achieve the desired outcomes? Is our program succeeding? When can we expect to see results? What conditions will influence failure or success? What other consequences can be anticipated as a result of our program? To answer each of these important questions, we need much better information, including accurate, real-time surveillance.

The right data will tell us how big a problem is, how well we are preventing and addressing it, and what else needs to be done. We have to be brutally honest with ourselves about the impact of our actions in order to move forward in the most productive manner. Eradication of bad public health management would likely save more lives than would eradication of any individual disease. These reforms can only occur if there is evidence to support their need.

Incorporating clinical data into public health information systems will improve program performance, as will information feedback loops to allow timely program modification. While increasingly common in the corporate world, using information in this way is still seldom done in the health field.

Improving surveillance to obtain better data to inform health action may not be the most exciting fix. It will never capture the imagination as new technologies can, though the latter often contribute to improving data collection and analysis. As the world becomes increasingly interconnected and interdependent, better information on disease patterns and program performance will become ever more essential to progress in global health.

Thomas R. Frieden is the Director of the US Centers for Disease Control and Prevention and former Commissioner of New York City's Health Department.

Chapter 36

Communicable Before Noncommunicable Diseases

LAURIE GARRETT

Investments in addressing noncommunicable diseases are being made at the expense of infectious disease control, which will have global repercussions if not addressed.

When the World Health Assembly convened in May 2013, the countries of the world responded to the World Health Organization's (WHO's) $1.2 billion budget deficit by slashing support for its communicable diseases programs (cut by 7.9%) and outbreak and crisis response capacities (chopped by an astounding 51.4%).

The following year when the Assembly reconvened, much of the floor debate concerned a new virus, Middle East Respiratory Syndrome (MERS), which was spreading in Saudi Arabia and several other countries. In the background, the smoldering Ebola outbreak in Guinea, Liberia, and Sierra Leone was hardly discussed. For both the MERS and Ebola outbreaks, the WHO's hands were tied, as the agency lacked sufficient resources to intervene with anything more than advice.

Three months after the 2014 World Health Assembly, the West African Ebola situation was out of control. It had spread from its initial Guinean origins to neighboring states, claiming three times more lives than any prior Ebola epidemic. Of course we all know how it continued to spread from there.

Interestingly, the same 2013 World Health Assembly that voted to nearly destroy the WHO's ability to respond to outbreaks and pandemics also chose to increase the agency's spending on noncommunicable diseases like diabetes and cancer by more than 20%. This figure doubles to 40% if you count increases for health promotion and systems development.

As the global health community races to target noncommunicable and chronic diseases, there is great danger that essential public health and infectious diseases response will suffer in a competitive budget climate. There ought not to be a tit for budgetary tat: building up noncommunicable disease capacity should never be at the expense of infectious diseases control and prevention as it was in May 2013.

In 2000, public health efforts—clean water, disease surveillance, food safety, and vaccination—garnered merely 1% of American health spending. Microbes do not disappear because a US surgeon-general declares victory over germs. The armamentarium of infectious diseases control is waning, and antimicrobial resistance is rising. The environmental conditions that foster animal-to-human disease transmission appear to be worsening, perhaps due to planetary climate change and loss of net terrestrial biodiversity.

Everywhere I travel around the world, I have asked doctors in clinical settings what they thought would bring the greatest benefit to the health of their people. Typically, new medical technologies and patented drugs rank high. It is on rare occasions that I have stumbled on morsels of wisdom. In Haiti, for example, a group of highly trained family physicians wanted to see the quarter of a million dollars an American medical school spent on their specialist training instead put toward repairing the water pumping and filtration system of Cap Haitian—the source of 90% of the illnesses they treat. In Ukraine a young medical microbiologist pleaded for basic diagnostic kits, even as his hospital administrator insisted the facility's primary exigency was a new cancer radiation therapy device. In Egypt physicians insisted they deserved the same high-tech tools in Cairo that they had been trained with in medical schools in the United Kingdom while refusing to even discuss the country's appalling nosocomial hepatitis C rate.

A decade ago Bill Gates invited me to sit in on a small meeting he had with three health ministers in Geneva. He told the ministers his foundation was prepared to help them, if they had wise plans for its funds. The first African minister asked for "a pile of laptops," with which to log health data on malaria. Gates turned her down, saying, "I am speaking of millions of dollars that can be a game-changer for the health of your people and you are asking for a few laptops?"

The second Asian minister said his country faced dire epidemics of lung and liver cancer, and requested financing for treatment centers. Gates responded by saying that tobacco use was astronomical in that Asian country, and given that the military was the major producer and commercial distributor of cigarettes, they needed to put a halt to that before asking for his support. As for liver cancer, Gates noted, inappropriate use of syringes fueled tandem epidemics of hepatitis B and C: he said "clean up the hospitals, stop reuse of syringes, and we can talk."

The third Latin American minister offered a detailed scheme for integrating infectious and chronic disease prevention campaigns at the community level, teaming public health and clinical practitioners in a united effort. Bill Gates grinned, clapped his hands together in a single sharp whack, and said, "Now that's something I can get excited about!"

As planning for the post-2015 development era draws to a close, talk of universal health coverage and noncommunicable diseases dominates. And that's just fine. But do not imagine for a moment that any country, regardless of its geography or GDP, can afford to build those capacities *at the expense of* classic public health and infectious diseases surveillance and control. We'll all regret it if they do.

Laurie Garrett is Senior Fellow for Global Health with the Council on Foreign Relations and winner of the Peabody, the Polk, and the Pulitzer awards for journalism.

Chapter 37

Human-Centered Design

MELINDA GATES

By understanding the problems that people face from their perspective instead of ours, we can design solutions that not only take root, but transform.

A few years ago in a rural part of East Africa, one of our foundation's grantees was having an unexpected problem: their treadle pumps were selling very well in some places yet very poorly in others. Treadle pumps help farmers irrigate small plots of land and turn a subsistent yield into a surplus they can sell.

Our grantee started tracking who was and who was not buying the pump—and soon learned that sales were slow because of how the pumps operated. Farmers had to stand on the pump and pedal, a movement that required a lot of hip swaying, similar to riding a bicycle. That presented a problem in communities where cultural norms considered women's hips swaying to be inappropriate. As long as the pump operated that way, most women farmers simply weren't going to buy it, no matter how useful or profitable it could be. But once the grantee realized the problem, the pump was redesigned, and adoption rates shot up.

This example illustrates a trend that makes me very optimistic about the future: the use of human-centered design principles to help people lead better lives.

At the most basic level, human-centered design is about listening. Organizations like our grantee go into communities to learn about the challenges people face and the realities of their lives. It's a process grounded in the understanding that the most valuable tools for improving people's lives aren't necessarily the ones designed in the shiniest labs; they are the ones people can and will actually use.

While this seems like a common-sense approach, the conventional wisdom among product designers going back decades was that if you could design a product that was sufficiently attractive and ingenious, people would want it, buy it, and shape their behavior around it. In the 1980s that began to change.

In part, that shift was driven by Donald Norman, a cognitive scientist at the University of California, San Diego. Everywhere he looked, Norman saw products that frustrated people: doors that were difficult to open, staplers that didn't staple, shower controls that seemed to require days of careful study to decipher.

Norman and his peers believed that people shouldn't have to adjust their behavior to products. Instead, it should work the other way around. Products should be adjusted to fit people's behavior. They coined the term "user-centered design," a concept that, coincidentally, rose to prominence about the time of the computer revolution. When I worked in marketing and software development at Microsoft, I saw firsthand how the needs of the customer informed the development of our products.

Today, the development community is starting to apply this same philosophy. In Ghana, for instance, it has driven amazing sanitation improvements. Where communities used to share a public toilet, residents complained about the difficulty of accessing them in the middle of the night. Now, companies have shifted to renting private toilets to individuals, to make them more accessible when they are most needed—and therefore, more likely to be used.

One of the most exciting aspects of this change is what it will mean for women and girls in developing countries. In many places, women and girls don't have a voice in society, so their needs are invisible and their preferences go ignored in their communities. As a result, the tools and solutions the global health community develops often don't reflect their needs or preferences either.

Bill and I started our foundation because we believe that every life has equal value, and we believe that everyone should have a voice in the conversations that will shape their future. Human-centered design helps ensure that these important conversations include everyone.

To cite one example I've seen over and over again, health clinics in many African countries will claim that they are well-stocked with contraceptives when, in fact, the only contraceptives they have available are condoms. That's a problem, because many women tell us that their partners won't agree to use condoms. For that reason, women prefer injectable forms of birth control. These injectable birth control methods last longer and are invisible, making them an effective way for women to protect their health and help better space their pregnancies—which we know benefits both them and their children.

This is a perfect example of the impact of human-centered design's power. On paper, condoms and injectables appear almost equally effective. But when we better understand the realities of these women's lives, we are able to design and deliver solutions that are more useful to them.

Putting women's needs front and center is especially important because women play a critical role in catalyzing global health and development: they are, themselves, agents of progress. When women like the farmers in East Africa are able to earn additional income, they invest in their children. When women are in charge of a household budget, they prioritize health, education, and nutritious food for the entire family. That means healthier, better educated children today—and healthier, more prosperous communities tomorrow.

The women I have met all over the world already have the potential to lift themselves out of poverty, to drive global development, and to improve global health. By helping women express their unique needs and preferences, human-centered design gives us all a means to unlock that potential.

Melinda Gates is Co-Chair of the Bill & Melinda Gates Foundation.

Chapter 38

A Data Revolution in Health

AMANDA GLASSMAN

Accurate, timely, and open health data matters for health impact, and modern technology makes data collection easier and cheaper than ever before.

After decades of rapid increases in health spending and technological advances, we should be able to unequivocally state the impact of health services on health status. Yet this is far from reality, across many different domains of global health.

Billions have been spent on malaria, yet we don't really know how many people die from the disease each year. Only 11% of developing countries have direct data on maternal mortality, and only a third of countries keep complete civil registries that capture deaths and causes of death. In sub-Saharan Africa, the United Nations estimates that only 7% of countries have more than 90% coverage of live birth registration.

Missing data is one challenge, but another is inaccuracy. Budgetary and donor schemes that tie funding to self-reported measures create incentives to overreport key data like vaccination rates or the number of kids in school. Without checks and balances to assure accuracy, our well-intentioned efforts to create rewards for progress can go horribly awry.

We also struggle to understand the relationship between our spending and what it produces. After 15 years and over $75 billion USD for

HIV/AIDS, we have only a vague idea of how much it costs to provide antiretroviral therapy for a year.

Finally, our data remains hidden. We don't publish our data sets and codes, our international agencies fail to report uncertainty intervals around their estimates, our disappointing clinical trials remain unpublished, and our prescription and utilization patterns remain unanalyzed.

Without this data, how can we assess our progress? How can we estimate needed resources? How can we be credible to ourselves and—most importantly—to the people who we have committed to keep healthy? How can we be accountable to parliaments and civil society organizations that count on data to track performance? How do we know if we are making a difference?

Accurate, timely, and open health data matters for health impact, and new technology makes data collection easier and cheaper than ever. Better data overall has been associated with improved governance and higher levels of foreign direct investment. It's time to harness this potential and revolutionize health data and its use.

Making progress in these areas will require willingness by all involved to experiment with new approaches that change the way data is collected, used, and made public. Here's how:

- *Fund more and fund differently.* Aid to support statistical systems in developing countries stands at less than 3% of total commitments. That means that donors don't spending enough on data, and countries don't make up the difference. Both need to recognize the magnitude of funding gaps, increase funding to national statistical systems, and create stronger incentives for improved data. Defining shared metrics for "good data"—that is accurate, timely, relevant, and available data—is a first step. Tying progress on those metrics to increased and flexible funding by experimenting with pay-for-performance agreements is a promising second step.
- *Build institutions that can produce and analyze accurate, unbiased data.* Many of the challenges surrounding data hinge on vulnerability to political and interest group influence, and

on a government's limited ability to attract and retain qualified staff. Governments should take steps to build capacity in production and utilization of data. This involves building data into policy and resource allocation processes, helping civil society and media organizations to access, analyze, and publicize policy-relevant data, and experimenting with new institutional models like public–private partnerships to improve collection and dissemination of data.

- *Prioritize the accuracy, timeliness, and availability of the core national health statistics* like births and deaths, and coverage, utilization, sickness, and safety. While we've benefited from the boom in household surveys on health, it's time to recognize that administrative data are as or more important for policy. These types of data are available more frequently and at levels of disaggregation that enable their use. Further, governments and donors can build greater quality-control mechanisms into the collection and analysis of data to avoid or manage the problems of over- or underreporting. This could be done through increased independent verification of core data, by embedding more explicit statistical support in line ministries (as is done in Côte d'Ivoire), or by requiring all data collection activities in health ministries be checked periodically by statisticians (as is done in Rwanda). National governments should also do more to encourage open data by releasing all nonconfidential, publishable data, including metadata, free of charge and online in a format that is analyzable and computer-friendly.

Taken together, these actions can build a solid foundation for a true data revolution.

Amanda Glassman is the Director of Global Health Policy at the Center for Global Development.

Chapter 39

Non-Drug Interventions Also Work

PAUL GLASZIOU

We are failing to capitalize on many non-drug therapies, which are often equally or more effective than their drug counterparts.

Imagine a drug that reduced by 70% the hospital readmissions and deaths for patients with chronic airways disease; or one that cut invasive melanoma rates by 50%; or prevented 50% of malaria cases; or prevented 50% of breech births? Doctors and patients would clamor for access, and companies would set high prices. These treatments exist but are neglected. They include exercise, daily sunscreen, insecticide-impregnated bed nets, and external cephalic version (turning the baby via the mother's abdominal wall). However, unlike their pharmaceutical brethren, non-drug treatments are less intensively researched, poorly described in that research, weakly regulated, and inadequately marketed—especially when cheap or free.

Non-drug treatments fall into several generic classes: exercise, diet, cognitive behavioral therapy, physical maneuvers, and a wide range of others. Perhaps the most neglected of them all is exercise for chronic illness—chronic lung disease, heart failure, cancer fatigue, diabetes, depression, and more. While exercise is often promoted as a preventative behavior in the healthy, the ill have the most to gain from physical activity. They are often fearful of exercise, as it can bring on symptoms such as breathlessness and fatigue, but, with persistence, it will improve function and quality of life, reduce relapses, and improve survival.

Certain exercises can also overcome functional deficits. Some of these are described in the popular book *The Brain that Changes Itself*, which highlights the discovery and impact of brain plasticity for rehabilitation. One clinical example is "mirror therapy"—where patients perform activities through feedback from a mirror—and it has been used to successfully treat phantom limb pain and regional pain syndromes after stroke.

So why are these effective interventions not used more often? Their neglect is partly because they are not aggregated into a respected compendium, equivalent to our pharmacopeias, which doctors look up when prescribing drugs. Instead these non-drug treatments are widely scattered in the burgeoning research literature and they are poorly described in current trials, which also creates problems in reviewing the evidence and making recommendations. Furthermore, there is no Food and Drug Administration equivalent to pass judgment on which of them are effective and which are not. More importantly, many of these non-drug interventions are cheap and have no patents, so there is no one to profit from their use other than the patient. Unlike pharmaceutical drugs, there is no company with a vested interest in marketing their benefits and encouraging their use. Ultimately, our neglect of effective non-drug treatments is a global market failure and it is our ethical obligation to correct it.

As a first step to addressing this gap, the Royal College of General Practitioners in Australia has begun to compile a handbook of effective non-drug interventions relevant to primary care. Such a compilation would also benefit lower-income countries, where resources and access are more constrained. In fact, many non-drug treatments, such as oral rehydration, solar sterilization of water, and insecticide-impregnated bed nets, are of most relevance in resource-poor settings.

We now need a global effort to extend this initiative to other disciplines and countries, so that these treatments can be tested, compiled, and promoted everywhere. Otherwise we risk wasting research dollars and efforts on expensive pharmaceuticals for conditions that can be treated with more affordable, and often more effective, non-drug interventions.

Paul Glasziou is Director of the Centre for Research in Evidence-Based Practice at Bond University and former Director of the Centre for Evidence-Based Medicine at the University of Oxford.

Chapter 40

Investing in Health Outcomes

TORE GODAL

Funding health system outputs, instead of inputs, is the smartest thing we can do for global health.

A transformational innovation is taking place in global health. Results-based financing, a pay-for-performance mechanism, is changing the way we think about health and development by linking incentives with results and funding only outputs and outcomes. For example, poor women are given cash when they can document that they have immunized their children, nourished them well, and sent them to school, or alternatively, that they have themselves attended clinics for pregnancy checks, delivery, or treatment of specific diseases such as HIV/AIDS. In addition, clinics and other health facilities receive financial bonuses based on the actual outputs they have achieved, measured by the number of deliveries performed or the quality of services provided.

This approach, which was first introduced in middle-income countries like Argentina, Brazil, and Mexico, is now being tested in large pilot projects in over 30 low-income countries, especially in sub-Saharan Africa and Asia.

The results are very encouraging. As little as 2%–5% of results-based financing in a health budget has given a much larger overall efficiency gain in health services, often on the order of 20%. A key enabler has been linking results-based financing to the World Bank's soft loans. Administrative overhead has been kept at 2% (because Bank staff carry out the work) and matching funds have multiplied investments (turning $429 million USD, as of April 2014, into $2.1 billion USD). This approach has the explicit approval of, and ownership by, the national ministries of finance that manage these programs.

For these reasons, results-based financing represents a smart investment not only because of its returns and leverage, but also in how it puts foreign aid on a distinct path to sustainable national financing in developing countries. Results-based financing platforms are now being joined on a country-by-country basis by other partners such the Global Fund to Fight AIDS, Tuberculosis, and Malaria, Gavi, and UNICEF.

Because results-based financing does not specify inputs but rather provides flexible funds, it has stimulated local innovation and decision-making. Experiences to date show that it puts the whole health system on a transformative path of reform. It also has the potential to contribute to a demand-driven, incentivized, and better aligned supply chain. Similarly, results-based financing management can be linked with electronic health-management information systems. As such, independent verification of data is possible and helps results-based financing to avoid overreporting of results.

In many areas, results-based financing is well-positioned to take us further from inputs to outputs and finally toward outcomes. For example, in the area of HIV/AIDs and other infectious diseases, we could shift our efforts from disease control to infection control through an epidemiology-based results-based financing approach. That would make a significant difference.

Tore Godal is a Special Adviser on Global Health with the Norwegian Ministry of Foreign Affairs and former Executive Secretary of the Global Alliance for Vaccines and Immunization.

Chapter 41

Imagining Global Health with Justice

LAWRENCE O. GOSTIN

If we imagine the aspiration of global health with justice, we would prioritize public health strategies—equitably distributed to the rich and poor alike.

The singular most transformative insight needed for better global health is that reductions in morbidity and premature mortality are not sufficient indicators of success if they come in the absence of equity. In other words, we can achieve high levels of global health but still lag in justice. To me this is unacceptable. What would constitute true transformation is achieving both overall population health *and* fair distribution of the benefits. We need global health married with justice.

But what would global health with justice look like?

First I can tell you what it wouldn't look like. Among the essential conditions for good health, too often we focus on health care. In doing so we take a narrow perspective, operating in silos—providing access to HIV/AIDS medicine here, reducing diarrheal disease there, tracking novel influenza viruses ad-hoc—rather than strengthening health systems. The immeasurable toll of injuries, mental illness, and noncommunicable diseases are too often underappreciated.

Does this tacit prioritization make sense given finite resources? I think not. Let me try to prove it to you by presenting a Rawlsian thought experiment.

Suppose—without knowing your life's circumstances (young/old, rich/poor, healthy/ill/disabled)—you were forced to choose between two stark options. The first option strongly prioritizes medicine: you could see a well-trained health-care professional whenever you want; attend the highest quality clinics and hospitals; and access the most advanced medicines and technologies. The second option strongly prioritizes public health: you would wake each morning with clean water to drink; fresh air to breathe; hygienic surroundings to enjoy; nourishing food to eat; an environment free from toxins, tobacco smoke, and malarial mosquitoes; and safety from preventable injuries and violence.

Blinded to your life's circumstances, there are compelling reasons for choosing the second option. The universal response to this experiment—whether in Beijing, Delhi, Kampala, or Washington, DC—is to choose public health. But that is the exact opposite of how global health is financed and delivered. This must change.

Investments in public health yield tremendous benefits. What is less often understood is that such investments will generally have the added benefit of promoting equity. When countries invest in genuinely public goods—water supply systems, sanitation, sewage, safe roads, vector abatement, pollution control, and the like—the benefits will, for the most part, accrue to rich and poor alike. The key point is that when government embeds healthy and safe conditions within the environment rather than allocating services to particular individuals or groups, then all human beings who live in that setting will benefit simply by the fact they inhabit the same space. This also requires additional work to ensure that the vulnerable gain the benefits, such as having their homes connected to water and sewage systems. This does not relieve society of the obligation to equitably allocate resources, but public health takes us down the path of justice.

Viewed in this way, the manifestations of justice in global health may look rather mundane. It will be evident in features of day-to-day life that are often taken for granted: the tap flowing clean water, the toilet flushing, the neighborhood market selling nourishing food, public sanitation controlling the spread of disease, and well-regulated industries. That is how I imagine global health with justice. Global health without justice is just not enough.

Lawrence O. Gostin is University Professor, Founding O'Neill Chair in Global Health Law, and Director of the O'Neill Institute for National and Global Health Law at Georgetown University.

Chapter 42

Putting People First

TEGUEST GUERMA

Community empowerment and participation is often neglected, but it is primordial for achieving better, cost-effective, equitable, and sustainable health for all.

Global health development, for all its increases in funding and attention, continues to follow an unfortunate top-down approach: policymakers, health leaders, and the international community at large presume to understand the universal needs of the poor—particularly the poor's most vulnerable and marginalized—and they design programs around these presumptions that are invariably a poor fit for the community they seek to help. Such initiatives are generally focused on prevention and treatment of a particular disease and often fail to incorporate more holistic approaches that address all forms of ill-health. Granted, our world is healthier than it's ever been, and the global community is investing more in health than ever before, but we could have achieved more for the money we've spent if there had been greater community empowerment and participation along the way.

Communities know their needs better than anyone else. Developing the skills and means to meet these needs enables them to create change from within and to improve their health in a sustainable manner. I strongly believe that communities must be an integral part of the solution. We should respect them, listen to them, and consider their views while developing any programs or projects around them. When communities are educated, mobilized, and empowered, they are motivated to improve their health-seeking behaviors. They will know the benefits of immunization, good nutrition, clean drinking water, and good hygiene. They will understand the importance of spacing their children and using bed nets, as well as the dangers of smoking and unprotected sex. With this knowledge and skill set they will be able to prevent many diseases, address the social determinants of their health, and change their lives in a sustainable way.

When communities are not participants in building solutions, they consider themselves external observers and view the project or program as belonging to the donor or the government—something imposed on them rather than something developed *with* them. For example, if a water site, clinic, or latrine built by an external organization is not functioning effectively, individuals living in that area are unlikely to care about its repair; it is not "theirs." On the other hand, empowered communities that are consulted and actively involved in the planning, implementation, monitoring, and evaluation of health projects will own and sustain these improvements. They will be accountable, and will in turn demand accountability from their leaders, for greater access to effective and quality health care, including the provision and training of skilled health workers. They will demand equity and make universal access for health a reality.

How can we facilitate this sort of community involvement and empowerment? By drawing and training community health workers from individual communities. These lay health workers must be trained and employed by the sponsoring health system to act as a bridge between community members and the health services being installed. Trained community health workers are able to carry out health promotion, lead education activities, and administer simple medical services while escalating complicated cases to a primary-level health facility. This strategy has allowed even the least-developed countries to make great progress in achieving some of the Millennium Development Goals with minimal resources. In Ethiopia, the training and employment of community health workers has produced impressive progress in maternal and child health: the number of maternal deaths per 100,000 live births was reduced from

990 to 460 between 2000 and 2013, and the mortality rate for children under 5 years old was reduced from 146 to 68 per 1,000 live births between 2000 and 2012.

I have personally witnessed the positive impact of involving and empowering communities in many areas where Amref Health Africa is currently working. In employing an inclusive approach, we have managed to stop female genital mutilation in sections of the Masai community in Kenya, where it has been practiced for centuries. We have also helped to reduce the incidence of malaria in the Afar communities in Ethiopia by working with community coordinators to introduce bed nets. Moving forward, we must channel the lessons learned from these successes into tackling both communicable and noncommunicable diseases in Africa. The failure to empower communities to practice healthy lifestyles has led to the proliferation of heart disease, cancer, and diabetes, creating immense health burdens. We have so far failed to do the right thing, and as a result these diseases have cost both money and lives.

Empowering and involving communities in whatever we do in health is imperative to achieving better health. We must ensure that doing this is given greater priority in order to achieve cost-effective, efficient, and sustainable health care for all.

Teguest Guerma is the former Director-General of Amref Health Africa and former Associate Director of the World Health Organization's HIV/AIDS Department.

Chapter 43

The Big Health Data Future

ANGEL GURRÍA

Health systems must imagine a future where big data is used to inform patients, providers, and governors, thereby improving quality and reducing costs.

An ugly truth within health systems is that the care you receive depends, to a great extent, on luck. Even in the best health systems in the world, recent work by the Organisation for Economic Co-operation and Development (OECD) shows that if you are fortunate enough to be born with a particular postcode, you can be two, three, even six times more likely to have a heart bypass than an individual born in another postcode within the same country. Startling as this may be, what is perhaps even more shocking is that we do not know what is causing this discrepancy. Are the high-intensity areas pushing unnecessary procedures on an unsuspecting population, or are there unmet needs in low-intensity areas? We don't know this because the people who run our health systems are expected to make critical decisions based on inadequate, fragmented, and paper-based information.

National health systems face a plethora of challenges, including enhancing fiscal sustainability, improving acute and primary care, and meeting the needs of an aging population. However, one of the greatest factors explaining the huge variation in the quality and intensity of care across countries and regions is the failure to manage health systems using evidence-based decision-making. This failure is very much related to the lack of reliable, comparable, and well-connected networks of big data, which are now essential for clinicians to deliver high quality medical services.

The big health data challenge has a myriad of manifestations and consequences. For example, in most developed countries, you will search in vain to find reliable comparisons of the quality of health care across different hospitals or physicians. There is—rightly—much talk about how patients should play a greater role in their care, but how can they when even basic information, like which provider to consult for their condition, is nonexistent?

Secondly, in most sectors of the economy, agents who provide excellent quality of service get paid more than those who are mediocre. In health, we usually either pay more to those who deliver more procedures or interventions, or we pay everyone the same regardless of the quality of the care they provide. Even in countries that claim to have pay-for-performance mechanisms, this usually translates into small bonuses for the best performers. The reason for these shortcomings is that we do not collate the metrics necessary to measure performance.

It is not that policymakers are unaware of these problems. Knowledge of variations in medical practice has been widespread since the 1930s. Few policymakers think that the way they pay providers is adequate, and disillusionment with clinical trials is widespread. The problem is that the data that quantify these discrepancies are not readily available in a form that can be used by decision-makers to inform and drive important policy changes. Indeed, no other area of the economy generates as much information as the health sector, and yet uses it so poorly.

Why is it that health systems are so poor at using data? One reason is that critical information is fragmented and disconnected, appearing in either hospital and medical records, disease and vital registries, or biobanks. Currently, only half of the 34 OECD countries have national policies addressing how data from electronic health records—which too are compiled by stitching together data from different sources—will be used to inform clinicians, monitor disease outbreaks, guide research, and improve patient safety. Furthermore, only half of OECD countries regularly use their existing health data sets to monitor health-care quality. Another challenge is that the use of patient health data is often blocked by well-intentioned legislation to protect their fundamental rights to privacy.

The potential benefits that better management of data could bring are enormous, and this lack of progress reflects a failure of the imagination. The range and volume of health data is growing exponentially and includes electronic patient records, administrative data, genetic data and biomarkers, and new streams of behavioral and environmental data from devices, apps, and social networks. Unfortunately, it all will sit unused in data warehouses unless fundamental changes are made. It is essential, for example, to promote proactive, engaged, and comprehensive data governance that enables data collection, sharing, and use without compromising patients' privacy. Stakeholders and the public need to be engaged in planning these governance arrangements and communication must be transparent. International sharing of data governance models will maximize global progress by helping all countries to move forward.

Making the most of the "big data future" in health care is the foundation upon which we can transform the quality and effectiveness of our health services. The OECD will continue to encourage global cooperation to ensure that data can be used to transform health care and citizens' rights to care and, ultimately, lead to better health-care policies for better lives.

Angel Gurría is the Secretary-General of the Organisation for Economic Co-operation and Development (OECD) and was previously Mexico's Minister of Finance and Minister of Foreign Affairs.

Chapter 44

Standing Up to Big Tobacco

JANE HALTON

Australia's success in cutting smoking rates shows we can and must act on many fronts at once to effectively tackle difficult public health challenges.

A single silver bullet solution to improve public health does not exist. Many public health challenges are driven by complex human behaviors which are not amenable to single measures or responses from the health sector alone. They demand action from multiple angles, with many measures implemented simultaneously within and outside the health sector, and require sustained action over time. Tobacco use is one such challenge. Australia has been able to mobilize sustained, multisectoral action to cut smoking rates. We can learn from this effort to address other public health challenges.

Tobacco use is responsible for around six million deaths and over half a trillion dollars in economic costs globally every year. It is also a leading risk factor for many noncommunicable diseases.

While smoking rates are declining in some countries, particularly in the developed world, the tobacco industry is expanding its markets in Asia, Latin America, and Africa. It has done so aggressively, by launching major marketing initiatives and issuing threats of legal action against governments considering tobacco control measures. This means that, globally, the deadly tobacco epidemic is still growing.

As a global community, we know what we need to do to decrease tobacco use. The Framework Convention on Tobacco Control provides a comprehensive road map of supply and demand reduction measures to be implemented inside and outside the health sector. It puts international law, and the power of international consensus, behind governments who take tobacco control measures.

Over the last 40 years, Australia has had a series of governments who have recognized the damaging effects of tobacco use on public health. Supported by an active and intelligent tobacco control movement in our NGO sector, governments at national and state levels identified and led the logical next steps and comprehensive approaches required to reduce this harmful habit. They have not allowed the tobacco industry to intimidate them, despite continued attempts by the industry to do just that.

Employing a series of measures including comprehensive advertising bans, social marketing campaigns, tobacco tax increases, smoke-free workplaces, health warnings, and quit lines, Australia halved its daily smoking rate among people aged 14 years or older from 30.5% in 1988 to 15.1% in 2010. Still, around 15,000 Australians continue to die each year from smoking.

Australian governments have redoubled their efforts to cut smoking rates. In 2010, tobacco excise tax was increased by 25%. New national social marketing campaigns were rolled out. "Tackling smoking" teams were deployed in indigenous communities. Smoke-free policies were extended to outdoor public spaces. And retail display bans were enacted.

In December 2013, Australia also took the world-first step of mandating plain packaging of tobacco products. This meant that packs were standardized in shape, in a color that was market-tested to be the least attractive to smokers, and with large graphic health warnings on the front and back. Smokers could no longer avoid the graphic health images or be distracted by the branding. People, especially young people, could no longer be misled by the attractive colors and shapes of packs into believing that some brands were less harmful than others, that the product was a status symbol, or that smoking was somehow glamorous.

The tobacco industry fought this change, and it fought hard. Plain packaging was challenged in Australia's highest court by four international tobacco giants, but the challenge was defeated and the measure was upheld. One company is challenging the measure under Australia's bilateral investment treaty with Hong Kong. Several countries, with tobacco industry support, are challenging the measure in the World Trade Organization. The Australian government is holding firm and fighting these challenges, insisting on its right to regulate to protect public health and to implement the Framework Convention on Tobacco Control.

Fearing that other countries will follow Australia's lead, the tobacco industry continues to try to sway international opinion by disputing the data about the effectiveness of plain packaging. Regardless, irrefutable evidence is emerging.

Tobacco clearances (the volume of tobacco products on which excise and customs duty is paid) in Australia fell by 3.4% in 2013 following the introduction of plain packaging in December 2012. Household expenditure on tobacco dropped to its lowest level ever in the March 2014 quarter. And daily smoking among Australians aged 14 years or older fell to a historic low: 12.8% in 2013 down from 15.1% in 2010. The decline in smoking rates is accelerating, and plain packaging is contributing to this record progress.

Australia's experience with tobacco control, including its plain packaging legislation, shows that governments can take effective, sustained, and multi-sectoral action to tackle the most difficult public health problems. It shows that standing up to Big Tobacco can deliver big results.

Jane Halton is the Secretary of Australia's Department of Finance and was previously Secretary of Australia's Department of Health, Chair of the World Health Organization's Executive Board, and Chair of the Organisation for Economic Co-operation and Development's Health Committee.

Chapter 45

Safe Food and Medical Products

MARGARET A. HAMBURG

Globalization has complicated how food and medicine are delivered; the task now is ensuring that these products remain safe.

Globalization—the rapid movement of people, products, and information across international borders—has been a buzzword for years. There have been countless debates about its benefits and disadvantages, as well as its relationship to and impact on inequality, inequity, health threats, and health outcomes. But often lost in this dialogue is the impact of globalization on two specific and essential components of global health: food safety and safe, high-quality medical products.

Globalization has fundamentally and irrevocably transformed the regulation of food and medical products. Ensuring the safety of the food we eat and the safety and efficacy of the medicines we use was, in the not so distant past, almost a completely unilateral function of national governments. Today, however, increasingly complex manufacturing, outsourcing, and supply chains have blurred the lines between domestic and foreign production, drastically increasing the opportunities for product contamination and adulteration. This makes food and medical product regulation a global health priority and a common challenge for all countries.

Consider the growing problem of food-borne illness caused by microbial, parasitic, and chemical contamination. Although disease-burden estimates are hampered by underreporting, some research attributes a considerable portion of the 2.2 million annual deaths from diarrheal diseases to food-product contamination.

Consider also the unacceptably high prevalence of substandard and falsified medical products that cause illness or death from toxicity, inadequate treatment, or drug resistance. Poor quality medicines erode the public's trust in medical interventions and threaten decades' worth of progress in combating infectious diseases such as HIV/AIDS, tuberculosis, and malaria. They also jeopardize our ability to prevent and treat noncommunicable diseases, the burden of which continues to rise dramatically. Such medicines pose a global threat, but they are felt most acutely in countries with high disease burdens and underdeveloped regulatory systems.

These examples demonstrate the need for strong regulatory systems capable of performing quality and safety oversight in the countries or regions in which food and medical products are manufactured, and through which they pass. Strong regulatory systems are essential to global health, safety, and security. They are the key to every country's strong and sustainable economic development and growth. Regulatory systems are also a linchpin to achieve accelerated progress toward the Millennium Development Goals, implementation of universal health coverage as envisioned for the future of international development, and mitigation of the growing dual burden of infectious and noncommunicable diseases.

One vision toward which the FDA has worked is the creation of a global product safety net maintained by relevant stakeholders, including governments, international organizations, industry, and academia, who cooperatively engage in core areas such as surveillance, reporting, inspection and compliance, and regulatory professional development. Cooperation is crucial in achieving this vision and enabling regulators to share information and best practices. Sustainable, cross-border, and multi-sectoral partnerships are also critical to addressing the challenges posed by globalization and the complexity of product supply chains, and to better positioning regulatory systems in the broader global health context.

A foundational milestone in these efforts was a resolution adopted by the World Health Assembly in 2014 on "Regulatory

System Strengthening for Medical Products." This resolution provides a framework for collective action and identifies priority areas for development, such as the collection and analysis of evidence and the implementation of science-based standards. Most importantly, it demonstrates that cooperation—coupled with commitment, flexibility, and resilience—can help regulators and their global health partners develop a shared set of goals and weave a global product safety net.

Margaret A. Hamburg is the Commissioner of the US Food and Drug Administration.

Chapter 46

Climate Change Is Here

KATHARINE HAYHOE

Addressing climate change is crucial for a healthy future.

We care about climate change because it exacerbates the challenges and problems we face today: access to clean water, plentiful food, reliable health care, and disease prevention. Failing to account for the ways climate change will affect global health puts people everywhere at risk in a very real and serious way.

We've known for a long time that there is an intimate linkage between *air pollution* and climate change. Climate change has already increased the number of deaths attributed to air pollution by a small fraction. Under a warmer climate, air pollution and its many health impacts—including asthma, respiratory disease, cardiovascular damage, and even premature death—will worsen if pollutant and precursor emissions are not significantly reduced.

We also know that *heat waves* cause heat exhaustion and heat stroke, as well as exacerbate the effects of allergies and preexisting illnesses. Risks disproportionately fall on the oldest and youngest members of society, as well as the infirm and those who lack the resources to protect themselves. Already, climate change has doubled the risk of heat waves such as occurred in Europe in 2003, which caused over 70,000 excess deaths. In some regions and over the shorter term, heat-related risks may be balanced by decreased risk from cold extremes. Over the long term and at the global scale, however, there is expected to be an overall increase in temperature-related illnesses and deaths due to extreme heat.

Climate also affects the transmission and geographic distribution of *disease*. Tracking potential impacts is complex: the spread of disease depends on the nature of the disease itself, the vector or carrier, and the many human factors that affect vulnerability and exposure, including socioeconomics and control measures. For example, a warmer climate might limit the dengue season in more equatorial locations by shortening the lifetime of the Asian tiger mosquito, but it might increase the risk at higher latitudes by expanding the mosquito season; however, the risk could be reduced if control strategies were implemented to reduce mosquito habitat.

As compelling as these direct impacts are, however, they represent only a fraction of the potential magnitude of the *indirect effects* of climate change on global health.

Climate change is altering the risk of both temperature and precipitation extremes. In some areas, it is increasing the risk of heavy rainfall or drought; in other areas, it is increasing the risk of both. Warmer ocean waters power stronger storms, and rising sea level increases the area inundated during those storms. Most insidious of all, climate change is shifting the long-term distribution and frequency of precipitation around the world, making wetter places wetter and dry places drier.

These indirect impacts can have potentially devastating effects on human security through their impacts on the availability of food, water, and other essential resources. Lack of resources can drive migration and large-scale exodus of refugees from affected areas, to the detriment of the health of both the displaced and the host people. Sea level rise alone may rob hundreds of millions of their homes within this century. Climate change may further act as a *threat multiplier*, increasing the risk of violent conflict or even plunging previously stable or marginal areas into failure. When states fail, public services, such as health, are among the first systems to be jettisoned in the fight for survival. The implications for global health and human society under such scenarios render first-world concerns regarding air pollution and urban heat waves nearly inconsequential in comparison.

Today, addressing global health without factoring in climate change is like pouring money, effort, goodwill, and prayer into a bucket with a hole in the bottom: a hole that is getting bigger and bigger with every ton of carbon emissions we spew into the atmosphere. That hole is climate change and it must be acknowledged and addressed for global health efforts to succeed. Tackling climate change is not a priority; it's a stark necessity for the well-being of humans on this planet.

Dr. Katharine Hayhoe is an atmospheric scientist, Associate Professor of Political Science, and Director of the Climate Science Center at Texas Tech University, and was lead author of the 2014 Third US National Climate Assessment.

Chapter 47

A Convenient Defense—Defining Affordability

DAVID L. HEYMANN

The global funds for vaccines and medicines, and the development model in general, require redefinition as demonstrated by issues such as the differing understanding of what is meant by "affordable."

Is a vaccine that protects children from meningitis in sub-Saharan Africa at 50 cents a dose affordable? No matter what we each may believe, affordability is a mutable concept. Much like the chameleon that changes color in different environments as a means of defense, the word *affordable* has different meanings in different settings, and has itself been used as a convenient defense.

The pioneering 50-cents-a-dose meningitis vaccine was the result of a successful transfer of the technology to an Indian vaccine manufacturer to develop a meningitis vaccine suitable and affordable for sub-Saharan Africa. Working with countries in sub-Saharan Africa, Gavi, the Vaccine Alliance, is now providing enough of this vaccine for most people below 21 years of age in 25 countries of the meningitis belt. The hope is not only to develop herd immunity in this population, but also to decrease nasal carriage—an added benefit of the new vaccine. However, countries with oil and mineral revenues in sub-Saharan Africa that have the capacity to purchase the vaccine have chosen instead to wait for Gavi to provide it.

Why are countries that can pay 50 cents a dose with their own financial resources waiting for Gavi to roll out the vaccines? Do these countries perceive the vaccine as unaffordable? Is 50 cents per dose still too high a price?

Questions such as these should reverberate throughout the development community when examining the current development model. They extend beyond vaccines and apply equally to medicines and innovative funding mechanisms such as the Global Fund to Fight AIDS, Tuberculosis, and Malaria. For example, antiretrovirals have become "more affordable" through the efforts of many countries and influential global health advocates to negotiate with the pharmaceutical industry. But for whom are they more affordable? Some middle-income countries have accepted the challenge of providing medicines from their own national budgets—which presumably means they now consider these medicines to be affordable. But others, some of which do perhaps have the resources to purchase these medicines, use "non-affordable" as a defense and a justification for not purchasing lifesaving vaccines as they await Global Fund allocations.

What will happen if funding for these lifesaving vaccines and medicines is no longer made available to countries that now rely on them? This is a realistic scenario. Gavi and the Global Fund may change the way they allocate resources or overall donor funding may decline. Co-financing—where countries provide a percentage of the cost when given development funding—is one short-term solution. Others advocate for a longer-term solution: a mandatory phase-in of national financing with complete assumption of costs as global financing is decreased. Given that countries clearly cannot be forced to buy medicines, however, the practicality of this approach is questionable.

So what is a true long-term vision and solution? What is the best definition of "affordable" when it comes to enabling all countries to procure lifesaving medicines and vaccines from their own national budgets? The short- and medium-term solutions are important; many have rightly fought for these innovative funding mechanisms and lives are being saved. But does the long-term definition of "affordable" go beyond different pricing for different markets and the application of flexibility in intellectual property and trade agreements?

Whatever the long-term definition of "affordable," it is urgent that we come up with it now as developed economies continue to falter and rapidly developing economies define their own roles in global health. It requires the focused willingness of all concerned—countries, industry, academics, international organizations, and advocates. And once we have that definition, it should never again be permitted to, like the chameleon, provide a convenient defense against the national allocation of resources for health.

David L. Heymann is Head and Senior Fellow of the Chatham House Centre for Global Health Security and Professor of Infectious Disease Epidemiology at the London School of Hygiene and Tropical Medicine.

Chapter 48

A Science of Global Strategy

STEVEN J. HOFFMAN

We must learn how to act collectively across national borders so that we can effectively address the transnational health threats and social inequalities that face us.

You might be surprised to read that cost-effective solutions already exist for many of the greatest global health challenges. It's true: we already know how to treat the 35 million people living with HIV/AIDS, prevent diarrhea that kills 760,000 children each year, and combat the health risks of alcohol, tobacco, and handguns.

Yet we face an exasperating gap between the health outcomes we can theoretically achieve and those we actually are achieving.

This gap is not caused by a lack of interest or investment; global health has never before received so much money or such prominence on political agendas. The real underlying problem is that our international system of sovereign states and decentralized control makes it very difficult for us to take collective action against transnational threats and common challenges. In the absence of a single global government, we still need effective global governance. Unfortunately, we do not do a very good job of making global decisions, coordinating responses, and enforcing rules. The consequences are serious: when countries do not work together or with non-state actors, it becomes difficult to contain the spread of infectious diseases, stop the flow of falsified medicines, finance the development of new antibiotics, reduce air pollution, or tackle the root causes of poverty.

Attempts to reform our global governance—to collectively address the health threats and social inequalities we now face—have proven difficult. This means that lightning-speed breakthroughs in biology and medicine have not been matched by the changes in global governance necessary to deliver on their promise. Despite a radically different landscape of greater transnational interconnectivity and interdependence, the basic tools of global governance have not advanced much since the Treaty of Westphalia codified state sovereignty in 1648. Confidence in these outdated tools, according to the World Economic Forum, is correspondingly at an all-time low.

There is no doubt that global governance failures can partly be attributed to the considerable time, resources, will, and support needed for reforms. But the other part is that we currently have insufficient knowledge about the reforms that can help achieve objectives that are sought, including the full range of legal, political, social, and economic strategies for global governance and collective action.

In other words, we know a lot about *what* we can do to improve global health, but we do not know *how* to organize ourselves across national borders to execute these needed actions.

A number of factors explain why knowledge of global strategy has lagged behind other fields. One is that few researchers with natural interests in global strategy—political scientists, sociologists, and legal scholars—have been trained in the empirical or big-data methodologies that can reveal deep insights beyond that of a curious human mind. A second is that such fundamental questions require interdisciplinary approaches that have not been supported by traditional academic institutions, incentives, or structures. A third factor is that research tends to be funded and conducted nationally, whereas expertise in this field is thinly spread across countries.

While global governance of the future is still to be imagined, trends like population growth, changing environments, and intensifying interconnectedness mean that we need new strategies for effectively managing transnational risks and for reaping each trend's possible rewards. Continued social progress and planetary survival depend on it. To be successful, these strategies will have to engage both state and non-state actors (because states alone have proven insufficient), promote mutual responsibility (because all must be invested in long-term success), and demand multidimensional accountability (because good intentions are not enough). My own research has shown the importance of having strategies that incorporate *incentives* for those with power to act on them, *institutions* designed to bring edicts into effect, and *interest groups* advocating domestic implementation.

The key questions in desperate need of answering, then, are which strategies can actually achieve global collective action, under what conditions, at what cost, and with what risks and trade-offs?

This requires three lines of social scientific inquiry. First, we need new approaches for synthesizing complex and conflicting evidence about when, how, and why different global strategies can facilitate collective action. Second, we must develop new analytical and empirical methods for evaluating global strategies and use them to draw novel insights about how to best design global initiatives, institutions, and interventions for maximal impact. Third, we need new ways to translate research into evidence-based collective action and train the next generation of strategic thinkers and leaders in these approaches and methods.

Working toward answering these important questions and pursuing these three lines of inquiry will help create a science of global strategy that gives global governors new tools to address the most pressing issues of our time. A healthy future depends on this ability to effectively work together and collectively solve the many overwhelming challenges we will all inevitably face.

Steven J. Hoffman is an Associate Professor of Law and Director of the Global Strategy Lab at the University of Ottawa and a Visiting Assistant Professor of Global Health at Harvard University.

Chapter 49

Time for Renewal

ARIANNA HUFFINGTON

Sleep, meditation, and mindfulness are performance-enhancing practices that help us lead more productive, engaged, and healthier lives.

We are living through an incredible time, when modern science is validating a lot of ancient wisdom. For far too long, we have been operating under the collective delusion that burning out is the necessary price to pay for accomplishment and success. Recent scientific findings make it clear that this couldn't be less true. Not only is there no trade-off between living a well-rounded life and high performance, but performance is actually improved when we include time for renewal, wisdom, wonder, and giving.

One study found that meditation can actually increase the thickness of the prefrontal cortex region of the brain and slow the thinning that occurs there as we age, impacting cognitive functions such as sensory and emotional processing. Dr. Richard Davidson, Professor of Psychiatry at the University of Wisconsin and a leading scholar on the impact of contemplative practices on the brain, used magnetic resonance imaging machines (MRIs) to study the brain activity of Tibetan monks. The studies, as Davidson put it, have illuminated for the first time the "further reaches of human plasticity and transformation." He calls meditation mental training: "What we found is that the trained mind, or brain, is physically different from the untrained one." And when our brain is changed, so is the way in which we experience the world. "Meditation is not just blissing out under a mango tree," says French Buddhist monk and molecular geneticist Matthieu Ricard. "It completely changes your brain and therefore changes what you are."

And this automatically changes how you respond to what is happening in your life, your level of stress, and your ability to tap into your wisdom when making decisions. "You don't learn to sail in stormy seas," Ricard says. "You go to a secluded place, not to avoid the world, but to avoid distractions until you build your strength and you can deal with anything. You don't box Muhammad Ali on day one."

The latest scientific findings have also confirmed the immense benefits of sleep. A 2013 study on mice showed that during sleep the brain clears out harmful waste proteins that build-up between its cells—a process that may reduce the risk of Alzheimer's. "It's like a dishwasher," said one of the study's authors, Maiken Nedergaard, Professor of Neurosurgery at the University of Rochester. Professor Nedergaard made an analogy to a house party: "You can either entertain the guests or clean up the house, but you can't really do both at the same time. . . . The brain only has limited energy at its disposal and it appears that it must choose between two different functional states—awake and aware or asleep and cleaning up." Far too many of us have been doing too much entertaining and not enough cleaning up.

A study published in *Science* even calculated that for the sleep deprived, an extra hour of sleep can do more for their daily happiness than a $60,000 raise. In fact, a number of studies have failed to find a consistent connection between extra money and happiness—as large increases of real income in the developed world over the past half century have not correlated with increases in reported happiness.

These findings make it clear that sleep, meditation, mindfulness, and renewal can no longer be seen as some sort of New Age escape from the world, vaguely flaky, definitely California. Rather, these are performance enhancers, practices that help us to be more productive, more engaged, healthier, and less stressed.

Arianna Huffington is the Chair, President, and Editor-in-Chief of the Huffington Post Media Group.

Chapter 50

Reliable, Unbiased, Reproducible Evidence

JOHN P. A. IOANNIDIS

Health decisions need to be informed by empirical evidence that is both transparent and reproducible.

Health decisions and policy have long been influenced, shaped, or dictated by academics and other experts, financially conflicted stakeholders (e.g., health-care and biopharmaceutical industries), ideologies and belief systems, and armies of pseudo-experts (e.g., mass media or politicians). Historically, empirical evidence has had a secondary role while these giants battled to control the territory of health. In the last few decades, evidence-based approaches have changed the landscape and empirical evidence has acquired a more pivotal role in this game. Randomized trials, large epidemiological cohort studies, meta-analyses, cost-effectiveness analyses, and evidence-based guidelines are prime examples of newly influential tools.

However, essentially little has changed. Evidence, in all forms and designs listed above, can still be influenced, shaped, or dictated. None of these designs are immune to bias, and all of them can be manipulated to serve the needs of people, corporations, or clubs that have strong allegiances and investments that favor specific types of results. The agenda, design, reporting, and interpretation of randomized trials can be tilted to serve specific answers that sponsors wish to extract. Epidemiological studies are subject to such extensive nontransparent exploration and data dredging that any desired result can be obtained. Meta-analyses that summarize biased studies further propagate the dominant paradigms. Cost-effectiveness analyses are notorious in their potential for manipulation of assumptions, models, and conclusions. Evidence-based guidelines include mostly recommendations for which either there is no evidence or there is biased evidence.

In this current state of affairs, how will we be able to generate reliable, unbiased, reproducible evidence on health? The answer to this question is not easy. In a sense, it is unlikely that there is a single simple answer. The fight between unbiasedness and bias is much like the one between antivirus software and computer viruses. We adopted all of these wonderful evidence-based designs to improve matters, and yet the old system found ways to circumvent them and to use them in its favor. We need to think of the next steps to address this challenge. This is likely to be an evolutionary, trial-and-error process, but a key theme will be increasing transparency in the research practices that generate evidence for better health.

For example, publication bias has long been a major problem for randomized trials. This happens when trials are not published—usually because they show negative, small, or otherwise uninteresting findings—leaving us with only sensational or extremely positive studies in the public domain. With the advent of trial registration, now we can at least know when trials are being planned and we can track which of them have been completed but not published. Still, this does not completely address selective reporting, given that registered trials may yet be published with distorted, selective approaches to their outcomes and results, offering a misguided picture.

This means that we need a new paradigm that is even more transparent—including more detailed, careful registration of the exact outcomes and of the full protocol, including statistical analysis plans. For epidemiological research, we are one step behind since not even registration has been widely adopted. Thus opportunities for free lunch abound. Wider raw data sharing will be helpful in improving the transparency of health-relevant research and would enable easier adoption of reproducibility checks to verify results. Changes in the reward and incentive system for biomedical research can help support research that is accurate, unbiased, and replicable over research that is seemingly novel, extravagant, and serves preconceived biases. In many fields, replication studies are considered to be uninteresting and of no value. A wider adoption of a replication culture, where results go through rigorous replication in independent data sets and studies, will help yield more trustworthy evidence. This transformation requires important changes in the peer review, funding, and publication systems.

None of these solutions are a panacea and several changes may need to be combined to have a substantial, durable effect on the reproducibility of health research. Moreover, one should always question and monitor whether specific solutions do indeed have the desired effects. Research practices that seem to work will need to be revisited periodically to ensure that no "viruses" have emerged for which new "antivirus software" is needed.

Unbiased reproducible research is unlikely to have a single silver bullet to solve all problems; it is, however, a step in the right direction. We need continuous questioning and some healthy skepticism. This is what science is supposed to do anyhow.

John P. A. Ioannidis holds the C. F. Rehnborg Chair in Disease Prevention at Stanford University and is a Professor of Medicine, Health Research and Policy, and Statistics, as well as Director of the Stanford Prevention Research Center and Co-Director of the Meta-Research Innovation Center at Stanford.

Chapter 51

Technology and Health Care in Africa

JAY IRELAND

Africa's health-care needs are changing, mobile digital technology is changing the game, local innovation is bringing modern health care to Africa, and the Industrial Internet holds new promise for the future.

Africa is very much on the rise. The continent has 11% of the world's population and sub-Saharan Africa hosts six of the ten fastest growing economies in the world. However, the continent also accounts for 24% of the world's disease burden and 1% of global health-care spending. Improving access, reliability, and affordability of health care will be significant drivers in realizing Africa's potential for rapid development.

Africa's health-care needs are changing. Communicable diseases remain the leading cause of death in Africa, but we are now also seeing a rise in noncommunicable diseases such as cancer, diabetes, and cardiovascular disease. Noncommunicable diseases are projected to account for 25% of all deaths in Africa by 2015, and by 2030 they are expected to surpass deaths from communicable disease. The ability to diagnose and treat these conditions is currently limited in many parts of the continent. Overall, access to quality health care is impeded by distance, inadequate infrastructure, and trained personnel. There is a dire need to extend the reach of services to rapidly growing urban centers and sprawling rural populations. Innovation and new technologies will play an important role in overcoming these challenges and transforming health care in Africa.

Fortunately, mobile digital technology is starting to change the game. The rapid penetration rate of mobile phone technology is increasing access to health care in Africa. Health workers at teleconsultation centers in remote African villages are using closed network mobile phones to speak with hospital staff and make treatment decisions. Regulatory agencies and pharmaceutical companies in Nigeria and Kenya are using mobile product authentication services to protect people from taking potentially harmful counterfeit drugs. Individuals can detect counterfeit medication by texting a scratched-off code to a secure number written on the package. Health workers are using SMS technology (short message service, aka texting) to transmit pre-delivery data to experts; early results show a 50% drop in infant mortality rates.

Local innovation is helping bring modern health care to Africa. In Tanzania, giant rats trained to sniff out tuberculosis in human sputum samples are evaluating 40 samples in 7 minutes, similar to a full day's output of a skilled lab technician. The Unjani Clinic-in-a-Box provides primary health-care services to underserved communities in South Africa for about $15 per consultation (including medicines). My company's Carestation 30 anesthesia-delivery system, developed with Kenyan doctors, is a modern but relatively inexpensive new technology with a six-hour battery to serve areas with low electricity supply. The Vscan, a pocket-sized mobile ultrasound battery-operated device, is providing physicians in remote areas with imaging capabilities. Combined with training of nurses and midwives to use these devices, ongoing projects in Ghana and Tanzania are demonstrating a meaningful impact on rural maternal and newborn health.

Availability of adequate financing is critical for local innovation to thrive. There is a need for better, more effective government funding along with creation of an attractive environment for venture capital and private investment. Localization is also critical. Companies must invest in local innovation capabilities and collaborate with African stakeholders to tailor innovation to local market needs.

The Industrial Internet—which refers to the integration of complex physical machinery with networked sensors and software—is moving the world to a new era of innovation and change. The Industrial Internet draws together fields such as machine learning, big data, and machine-to-machine communication to ingest data from machines, analyze it (often in real time), and use it to adjust operations. This merging of the digital world with the world of machines holds the potential to transform global industry. The global health-care industry is a prime sector for Industrial Internet adoption because of the strong imperatives to reduce costs and improve performance—enabling safe and efficient operations. It is estimated that the Industrial Internet can drive global health-care costs down by about $100 billion a year, making health care more affordable to people.

In addition to improved medical efficiencies, the digitization of health care holds the promise of fewer medical errors, improved quality of life, and actual saving of lives around the globe. Medical equipment can be monitored, remotely controlled, and automated to provide quality care to homebound patients and people in remote areas. The Industrial Internet will further facilitate access by enabling, capturing, and transferring knowledge easily between people, systems, and sites.

Africa's health-care sector could look very different over the next decade. In terms of technology access, we could start to see a greater level of public awareness and self-diagnosis, while mobile technologies will continue to improve access within the health sector. And with adoption of the Industrial Internet, we should start to see borderless diagnostics and treatment decisions that increasingly transform health care in Africa.

To realize its potential, Africa requires better-equipped facilities, more highly trained health-care professionals, adequate financing, and close collaboration between the private sector and government.

Jay Ireland is the President and CEO of GE Africa, former President of GE Asset Management, and former President of NBC Universal Television Stations and Network Operations.

Chapter 52

Love Is the Cure

ELTON JOHN

More than science, training, infrastructure, or education, public health is first about compassion and dignity.

I have some good news. The single biggest change that is needed now, the one that could most radically improve our health-care systems, is free. It can't be patented by any corporation. It doesn't eat into anybody's budget.

What we need most is compassion.

I know that might sound, at first glance, airy-fairy or wishy-washy, but I mean it quite literally. I know it's true because compassion saved my life, and there is now significant scientific evidence that it can save millions more.

When I was in rehab, after hitting the rock bottom of my drug addiction, they taught me that "your secrets make you sick." All the years of shame—for being gay—had caught up with me. By showing me love and compassion, they taught me—slowly, carefully—how to show it to myself. If I hadn't confronted that stigma, I don't think I would have survived to write this.

Last year, I met a young Ugandan woman who was living in Britain, who I'll call Waangari. When she was sixteen, she was raped by her brother-in-law. She knew it would devastate her sister, so she never told a soul: instead, she just sank into shame. She later married a man who took her to Britain, where he began to beat her up all the time. Alone and knowing no one, she fled to a refuge and was told at a medical checkup that she was both pregnant and HIV-positive. When she went for treatment, the nurse in the antenatal ward looked at her notes and told Waangari that she could not bathe on hospital property "because of your condition." She tried to argue, but the nurse called a meeting and told all the nursing staff on the ward that Waangari had to be kept in a separate single room away from the rest of the patients, and confined only to showers. She started having flashbacks to the shame of being raped and infected with HIV in the first place—and it was so unbearable that she stopped going to her checkups, or for treatment.

By denying Waangari compassion—indeed, by showing her contempt—that health-care provider risked causing a chain reaction. Waangari could have gotten sick; her baby could have gotten sick; and either of them could have later passed on the HIV virus to others, who could have passed it on to others, and so on. The potential human, financial, and medical cost of the nurse's contempt is incalculable, yet scenarios like this are playing out every day, all over the world, today.

Waangari got lucky. A few months later, her general practitioner apologized when she heard this story and arranged for an obstetrician to meet her at the hospital bus stop and hold her hand as they walked onto the ward. Waangari was so moved by this act of compassion that, after her child was born, she started to train as a nurse. Today, she is showing compassion and love every day to her own patients.

The virus of kindness infected Waangari; it is now radiating out from her, and it is beating the HIV virus. I have heard stories just like hers at projects funded by my foundation in Russia, Ukraine, South Africa, and Washington, DC. Too often, doctors have looked into the eyes of these people, and seen not a human being with feelings and needs like their own, but only a deadly virus. By doing this, they have made the virus ever more deadly.

We will only end AIDS if we end these stigmas—toward people with HIV, toward gay people, toward drug users. Many will not come forward to be tested and treated if the cost is being sneered at and shamed. For people who already feel a great deal of shame—because of their sexuality, drug use, or sex work—even a cold glance can be enough to trigger an internal spiral of shame that will drive them out the door and out of the reach of medical intervention.

This insight goes much further than AIDS. As Dr. Tom Shakespeare, a British sociologist who has studied this topic, highlights, hospitals in the British National Health Service that showed lower levels of compassion to patients led to higher death rates across the board. Yet he explains that one medical consultant had shrugged, "I find the ward round goes much faster if you don't talk to the patients."

Compassion saved my life when I was sick. It saved Waangari's life and it led her to save the lives of others. I have seen compassionate doctors and nurses saving thousands of people across the world. They know medicine is not offered to machines. It is not like the petrol we pump into our cars. It is offered to human beings—with dreams, despairs, and desires. It costs nothing to remember this, but it means everything.

Elton John is an Academy, Grammy, and Golden Globe Award–winning musician and Founder of the Elton John AIDS Foundation.

Chapter 53

Multi-Sectoral Investments for Health

MUSTAPHA SIDIKI KALOKO

Substantially reducing the world's disease burden and improving health overall requires an expansion of our investments to sectors outside of health.

Disease is not only a problem of health, but also a persisting impediment to development. Over the last two decades, billions of dollars have been disbursed, especially to the developing world, to support disease control programs and health research. Despite all of these investments, health still remains a huge burden in both the developed and developing worlds, leaving most countries unable to meet the Millennium Development Goals.

Perhaps we should be investing our resources differently. Perhaps we are too focused on funding direct health interventions and ignoring other crucial areas of human life that could act as vehicles to good health.

As we formulate the post-2015 agenda for the future of international development, we must recognize that investing in health alone has not produced the results we want to see. However, it has been shown that an investment in health coupled with a corresponding investment outside of health can produce positive results.

Malaria eradication is one such example. Efforts to control the disease were accompanied by investments in modifying the environment and improving economic conditions. Though these collateral investments may not have been targeted at malaria control, evidence shows that investing in the social determinants of health was the key to success against the deadly disease. If we are to make meaningful progress in global health, this same approach must be applied to all health interventions.

To begin, the world should embrace universal health coverage and co-invest in its enablers. Universal health coverage is important because it reduces the gap between social classes by ensuring that everyone gets the health services they require without suffering fiscal hardship when paying for them. Successful implementation of universal health coverage requires a strong, efficient, well-run health system; a system for financing health services; access to essential medicines and technologies; and a sufficient capacity of well-trained, motivated health workers.

These conditions cannot be met by investing in health alone, and require corresponding investments outside of health. Although universal health coverage is now receiving substantial worldwide attention, the focus is on improving health financing systems with few complementary efforts in other sectors. The operationalization of universal health coverage needs to look at physical and financial barriers to access both within and beyond the health system.

Effective universal health coverage requires systems that mobilize the bulk of funds through prepayment, such as taxes and insurance. They must later pool these funds to spread the financial risk of illness across the population. Such systems almost always lie outside the health sector, and others, such as insurance, could even be outside the public sector. Investments into the health sector coupled with investments to strengthen tax authorities or insurance systems would be a significant contribution to universal health coverage and better health. Systems that strongly support social protection have been known to lead to better quality care.

Investment in infrastructure can improve access to health care by creating jobs that enable people to pay for health services. It modifies the physical environment, leading to better housing, safer roads, and cleaner water and sanitation systems. All of these changes contribute to improved livelihoods, healthier people, and a decreased demand for health services.

Equally, investment in education holds immense benefits for health. General literacy is an important determinant of health and is particularly significant in the success of health promotion initiatives. Educated individuals are less likely to engage in behaviors that are detrimental to good health, and more likely to undertake preventative measures to avoid health risks.

Partnerships with the media can also be advantageous, as they are well-placed to promote public health goals. Leveraging media advocacy can also drive policy change and move the public health discussion from individual health behaviors to macro-level changes in the way health care is governed and delivered.

Lastly, we must invest in better law enforcement. Globally and nationally, we have many laws that support the right to health and access to health care. These include laws that address illegal prescriptions and counterfeit drugs, protect mental health patients, and prohibit insurers' use of generic information in pricing, issuing, or structuring health insurance. Unfortunately, in most places, especially in the developing world, enforcement of such laws remains difficult. This has resulted in major costs to health in the form of severe human rights violations, faulty medicines, and heavier disease burdens. Although law enforcement often lies outside the health sector, co-investment in this realm will provide another avenue through which health can be improved.

Substantially reducing the world's disease burden and improving health overall requires an expansion of our investments outside of the health sector. Health is influenced by many other determinants, including infrastructure, education, economic status, and law enforcement, and accordingly our approach to better health must be multi-sectoral. If we are to see significant advancements in global health within our lifetimes, each dollar invested in the health sector should be coupled with at least another dollar in a corresponding sector.

Mustapha Sidiki Kaloko is the Commissioner for Social Affairs of the African Union.

Chapter 54

Secondary Schooling for Girls

ANGÉLIQUE KIDJO

If we want to see sustainable change in health in developing countries, we need to provide girls and young women with access to secondary education.

I was born and raised in Benin, West Africa. Even though my continent is still perceived only as a land of poverty, war, and disease, I have to say I had quite a great childhood. And I have been able to accomplish my childhood dream: to be a singer and to travel the whole world. It is true that I was very lucky, not because I was born into a rich family—my dad worked at the post office—nor because I was discovered at a young age by some powerful music mogul. The reason for my success story? My mother was educated and understood the importance of good health and vaccination. Her high school education allowed her to follow correctly the advice of doctors and to go beyond the superstitions that prevent many parents from vaccinating their children.

A memory from my childhood that I will always remember is the blue UNICEF truck roaming the streets, scaring me. Mom would give us no choice: we had to get our shots and I hated needles. I would run away and hide, but she would always find me and make sure my vaccinations were up to date. She had a big medical book called "Mon Médecin" (My Doctor) that described all the organs and diseases known at the time. All of us brothers and sisters would avidly read it. We learned the importance of proper hygiene, nutrition, and care, and we all benefited from this knowledge over the span of our lives.

I didn't realize it at the time, but my mother was the exception and not the rule. As a UNICEF Goodwill Ambassador, I have participated in many health campaigns and the biggest challenge I've found is that, often, the health message we are trying to convey is not properly understood because of a lack of education among mothers. They want the best for their children. They have amazing strength and great patience. But the complexity of diseases like HIV/AIDS, as well as the strict necessity of prevention, are unclear to many of them. A lot of traditions, rumors, and fears run contrary to what seems like common sense in the Western world. Moreover, certain communities don't speak the main language of the country, rendering public service announcements useless. There is only so much that campaigning can do if the message itself is not fully understood.

The Millennium Development Goals brought incredible attention to the importance of primary education for both girls and boys. But I think the level of education required to understand complex health information extends beyond primary school. Girls, who will in turn become mothers, need access to a more sophisticated schooling system if we want them to implement all the available measures that will save lives. It won't be easy to attain. There is a lot of pressure on teenage girls to do other things beside going to secondary school, including getting married, caring for newborn babies in their families, or attending to their homes when their mothers are away. That is why secondary education for girls is the best investment we can make. Equipped with the additional knowledge and skills they will gain, girls will be able to accomplish their dreams.

I want every young girl in Africa to have the same opportunities as I did!

Angélique Kidjo is a Grammy Award–winning Beninese singer-songwriter, UNICEF Goodwill Ambassador, and Founder of the Batonga Foundation.

Chapter 55

Getting Health Delivery Right

JIM YONG KIM

Better health-care delivery will save millions of lives, but this requires bridging the gap between knowledge and implementation.

How do we get health-care delivery right in developing countries?

Finding the answer is urgent: in 2012 alone, over 6 million children under age 5 died—that is nearly 18,000 children every day. More than 1 billion people do not have access to health care and 100 million fall into poverty each year because of out-of-pocket health-care expenditures.

Scarce public financial resources, whether from developing countries' budgets or donor funds, must be used effectively and efficiently. Donors and governments want real value produced for their financial investments, and we should assess this value comprehensively to show its true impact. Unfortunately, health data are often of poor quality or unavailable; many health delivery systems are designed in an ad hoc manner to address one health problem among many; and best practices spread too slowly.

Yet evidence shows that smart investments will not only save lives but also improve the health and prosperity of millions, especially the extreme poor. In fact, nearly a quarter of the income growth in low- and middle-income countries between 2000 and 2011 has been attributed to better health outcomes.

Effective health-care delivery will involve using a more rigorous and systematic approach to outcomes and how to achieve them. It will require sustained focus and efforts to develop what some of us have called "health-care delivery science." This new approach includes five elements.

First, we need to support frontline implementation by collecting local experience and then feeding that knowledge back into practice. To build a health-care delivery science, we need a clearinghouse of information about program design, best practices, synergies, policy constraints, environmental determinants, and other elements of global health-care delivery. The collection of data should run seamlessly from bedside to seminar room and back to the field, enabling joint problem-solving, and linking local action to global evidence.

Second, we must teach the skills that are relevant for effective delivery, based on the experience of the most successful practitioners. Several years ago I was part of a research and teaching program called the Global Health Delivery Project, which aimed to help fill this gap between policy, research, training, and delivery in settings of poverty. A substantial body of open-source case studies examining care delivery in response to various diseases has been developed, and a family of complementary courses is being taught at Harvard University, Dartmouth College, Columbia University, and by the Ministry of Health and other partners in Rwanda.

Third, we need to increase investments in health-care delivery systems, both public and private, to ensure access to high-quality services. Many health-care delivery systems suffer from underinvestment in basic infrastructure, essential inputs, and key systems. Investments that can improve supply chains, information management, inventory controls, and accounting systems can yield large returns on performance in low-resource environments. In addition, addressing barriers to access, especially for the poor and marginalized, will ensure equity and reduce disparities.

Fourth, we must undertake implementation research to spur innovation and evaluate new interventions. Opportunities for study and research—along with the funding to support them—are steadily increasing. Universities, teaching hospitals, and other health-care institutions can engage this agenda in new ways and develop frameworks, knowledge, and practices that will benefit patients and practitioners.

Fifth, we need to develop new theoretical and analytical frameworks that can help explain and adapt successful approaches to solving delivery problems. The future of health-care delivery science lies in bringing new disciplines, perspectives, and methodologies to bear on the challenges at hand.

Combining these five elements will help us understand the full complexity of building health systems and delivering care, especially in resource-poor settings. It will take time to create, and like any science, it will never really be complete. Donors should channel resources to the most successful approaches, and work with governments to build a supportive public policy environment.

The goal is not just to deliver health-care services, but rather to achieve a healthier global population and reduce health disparities. A rigorous health-care delivery science offers a promising path to reduce poverty and improve health for all members of the human community.

Jim Yong Kim is President of the World Bank Group and former President of Dartmouth College.

Chapter 56

Closing the Pain Divide

FELICIA MARIE KNAUL

Uneven access to basic pain medications is a glaring symptom of the many health inequities we continue to face.

The world is plagued by a pain divide that impoverishes efforts to reduce human suffering. It is both a cause and effect of other social and health inequities.

The statistics are mind-boggling and horrifying. The World Health Organization estimates that every year tens of millions of people—including 5.5 million terminal cancer patients and 1 million end-stage HIV/AIDS patients—suffer needlessly in severe pain because they do not have access to pain medications. Globally, some 5 billion people—the vast majority of the world population—live in countries with little or no access to opioid analgesics.

The distribution of access to pain control is grossly inequitable. In all but the highest income countries of our world, access is shockingly low. Data from Treat the Pain show that the poorest 10% of the world's population live in countries where less than 200 milligrams of morphine (or equivalents) are available per death from HIV or cancer. The figures are only marginally better in middle-income countries. By comparison, the richest 10% of the world has access to almost 100,000 milligrams and the United States and Canada close to 350,000 milligrams.

The need for access to pain medications is ubiquitous and universal. There are only two moments that are experienced by all human beings: birth and death. Both are moments when safety and security should be paramount, and where health systems have a key role to play.

Despite the universality of need—100% of people die—global health is marked by a dearth of motivation, metrics, money and means to close the pain divide and provide for safe and secure death and dying and palliation of suffering. Priority-setting and values that guide the investment decisions that are taken by health policymakers focus on extending or improving quality of life, often with a particular concern for increasing labor market productivity. Dignity in dying and pain control score near zero in these measures, despite the fact that most individuals, when asked, highly value avoidance of pain.

Indeed, the universality of the need for pain control and palliative care is, ironically, at the epicenter of why this area has been neglected in global health. These interventions are not specific to a disease, although cancer is most often associated with the need for pain control. This fact, combined with the almost ubiquitous fear of death and focus on extending life, has limited the advocacy and health resources devoted to this cause.

Yet pain control should be an issue around which all disciplines and disease groupings can unite. Solving the problems of access for one disease implies solutions for all diseases. Further, pain control constitutes an exemplary diagonal strategy (a synergy between disease-specific and broad-based health system interventions) that provides positive externalities. For example, surgery—which embodies interventions necessary at all stages of the life cycle—relies heavily on the need to control acute pain.

Closing the pain divide is an equity, health, and human rights imperative that can be addressed at low cost and in ways that broadly strengthen health systems in low- and middle-income countries. Pain medications, primarily medicinal opioids, have been proven to be cheap, effective, and feasible to administer even in the poorest countries. Access to medications can be significantly improved by correcting restrictive and cumbersome national and global legislation and regulation that tends to unnecessarily inflate prices well beyond the actual cost of producing and delivering the drug.

There are ways to close the pain divide; what has been lacking in global health is the will to do it. A combination of advocacy-inspired evidence and evidence-based advocacy applied to policy can and will provide solutions. Indeed, we are already seeing this remedy breathe into palliative care in several low- and middle-income countries. These lessons must be documented, disseminated, drawn upon, and dispensed.

Felicia Marie Knaul is Director of the Harvard Global Equity Initiative, Associate Professor of Global Health and Social Medicine at Harvard Medical School, and Founding President of the Mexican nonprofit organization Tómatelo a Pecho.

Chapter 57

Equity in Child Survival

ANTHONY LAKE

If we addressed inequities in child survival, all children would have a similar chance of surviving until their fifth birthday—no matter where they live.

Imagine if every person who wanted better health care could stand up and demand it. Imagine if all citizens had the tools to help their governments better identify where health services are most needed and to hold leaders accountable for delivering them.

We don't have to imagine. In Uganda, a free SMS-based (text message) service called U-report lets nearly a quarter million youth across the country speak out about issues that affect them and report which services are working and which are not.

In every part of the world, dynamic partnerships are expanding health services, reaching more children and families. Over the past 20 years we have driven down the cost and steadied the supply of essential health products. Thanks to innovative financing and new ways of delivering vaccines, global immunization is at an all-time high, with 440 million children and adults reached. Collectively we have almost halved the number of deaths among children under 5 since 1990. At the rates of reduction now being experienced in Bangladesh and Rwanda, almost every country in the world could bring its child mortality rate to below 20 per 1,000 by 2035, converging with rates achieved in high-income countries.

Failure to identify and address inequity is the greatest barrier to achieving this goal. We have to do more than improve our delivery of services. To reach every child, we need even more focus on enhancing the capacity of children and families to take advantage of quality health services.

Community engagement and practical policy measures can make a real difference in promoting health equity. Where financial barriers impede access, cash transfers can offer part of a solution. Where cultural barriers exist, governments, civil society, UN agencies, and faith-based leaders can join together to overcome mistrust. In polio endemic countries, for example, partners have organized mass communication efforts to educate parents about the risks of polio and the benefits of the vaccine. Of the households reached by polio workers, only 0.6% refused the vaccine. And increasingly, polio outreach is part of integrated packages of health services, so that children are not only protected against polio, but they are also reached by other lifesaving vaccines and nutrition interventions.

Where the barriers are geographical, community health workers are bridging the gap between families and health-care facilities. In Ethiopia, a health extension program has trained and employed more than 30,000 community health workers. This has contributed to Ethiopia's achieving the Millennium Development Goal of reducing its under-5 mortality rate by two-thirds—three years ahead of deadline.

But to continue bending the curve, and to reach the children who are consistently excluded, we will need to go beyond health.

Birth registration is a child's passport to vital public health-care services, education, and social security. Yet nearly half of all children under 5 worldwide lack birth certificates—and it is the poorest and most marginalized who are least likely to be registered. Today, health workers are registering newborns with a simple text message sent from a basic mobile phone. The technology is not innovative, but using it for free and for universal birth registration is.

Another key intervention is nutrition. The latest science shows that the keystone to building a more equitable world may lie within every child. A child's brain grows fastest during the earliest days of life: between 50% and 75% of an infant's energy is spent on brain development. So nutrition is extremely important to support growth and connectivity of brain cells and full cognitive capacity.

In 2014, we celebrated the 25th anniversary of the Convention on the Rights of the Child: a nearly universally shared and legally binding commitment to help every child fully realize her rights, including the right to health. In 25 years we have made progress toward the Convention's vision of a world fit for every child, but we have so much more to do.

Some 18,000 children under 5 die every day—mostly from preventable causes. These children live and die in the poorest, most dangerous, and hardest to reach areas of every country. In most cases, their deaths are preventable. And in most cases, their families and communities are invisible within the national averages we use to measure development progress.

As long as any child is excluded, we are not living in the world we imagine. As we work on behalf of the rights of all children, everywhere, we must challenge ourselves to be bolder, quicker, more creative, and ever more innovative—just as children are as they grow.

Anthony Lake is the Executive Director of the United Nations Children's Fund (UNICEF).

Chapter 58

Evidence-Informed Health Systems

JOHN N. LAVIS

Citizens and other key stakeholders, informed by the best-available data and research evidence, are best positioned to pick and operationalize the ideas that can iteratively strengthen health systems.

Strong health systems are needed to get the right mix of cost-effective programs, services, and drugs to those who most need them. Academic journals, books, news outlets, and the Internet are full of ideas about how to strengthen health systems. But how can we pick and operationalize the ideas that can take a given health system from where it is now to where it should be? And how can we continue doing so iteratively as new challenges arise, competing ideas emerge, and health and political systems evolve?

It's sexy to focus on the latest ideas for what we need to do. At any given moment, you can find someone calling for increasing the scope of practice for nurses and other health professionals so that they can deliver needed care in underserved areas. Others call for the introduction of pay-for-performance schemes to improve the performance or efficiency of health providers. Still others call for centralizing many types of procedures in high-volume facilities to improve quality and achieve better health outcomes. The list of called-for changes to health-system arrangements is nearly endless.

Who should we listen to?

One part of the answer is informed citizens. Citizen panels—a form of deliberative dialogue—are an approach to systematically soliciting the values and preferences that citizens believe should drive particular decisions about their health system. A citizen brief can synthesize the best-available data and research evidence about a pressing challenge, options for addressing the challenge, and key implementation considerations. Informed by this brief, an ethnoculturally and socioeconomically diverse group of citizens can, with appropriate facilitation, work through the challenge, options, and implementation considerations and arrive at an informed judgment. If we want *people-centered* health systems, those elected or hired to make tough decisions about a given system need to listen to those who the system is meant to serve.

The second part of the answer is informed policymakers, managers, professionals, and civil society representatives. Stakeholder dialogues—again, a form of deliberative dialogue—are an approach to systematically soliciting the tacit knowledge, views, and experiences of those who understand how a given health and political system really works and what it takes to make change happen. Like a citizen brief, an evidence brief can synthesize the best available data and research evidence about a pressing challenge, options for addressing the challenge, and key implementation considerations. Informed by this brief, a purposively selected group of individuals—who both bring unique insights to the table and can champion change among unique constituencies based on what they learn—can work through the challenge, options, implementation considerations, and next steps for different constituencies. If we want *high-performing* people-centered health systems, we need to listen to those who understand the institutional constraints, interest-group dynamics, values and preferences, and "outside" influences operating in the political system where decisions are going to be made, and who understand the governance, financial and delivery arrangements operating in the health system where those decisions are going to be implemented.

We've come a long way in being able to synthesize the many types of data and research evidence needed to inform these deliberations. For example, Health Systems Evidence makes available all synthesized research evidence and economic evaluations about health systems in a database that can be searched in seven different languages (www.healthsystemsevidence.org). We've also come a long way in being able to prepare citizen and evidence briefs and convene deliberative dialogues. Evidence-Informed Policy Networks (EVIPNet) are undertaking such work in a broad range of low- and middle-income countries, and their briefs and dialogues have been shown to be highly useful to key policymakers and stakeholders, to lead to strong intentions to act on what was learned, and to translate into concrete changes in policy and practice.

But we still have a long way to go. Health Systems Evidence is used by nearly 10,000 health-system policymakers and other stakeholders around the world. It needs to be used by hundreds of thousands. EVIPNet is active in a few dozen countries, but it needs to be institutionalized in these countries and its approaches adopted in many others. The World Health Organization continues to use a clinical paradigm for creating one-size-fits-all health-systems guidance, but it needs to be preparing accompanying workbooks that support countries to contextualize the guidance for their unique health and political systems through briefs and dialogues, among other approaches.

It's not sexy to focus on *how* questions—in this case, how can we pick and operationalize the ideas that will iteratively strengthen health systems. But this particular how question needs to be answered if our focus is long-term gains in global health, not short-term wins for best new idea. Citizen panels and stakeholder dialogues, informed by the best-available data and research evidence, are my answer.

John N. Lavis is Director of the McMaster Health Forum, Professor of Clinical Epidemiology and Biostatistics at McMaster University, and Adjunct Professor of Global Health at the Harvard T.H. Chan School of Public Health.

Chapter 59

Ignorance about Causes of Death

ALAN LOPEZ

We need better data about changing cause-of-death patterns among adults in developing populations and improved monitoring of adult survival.

Information may well be power, as is often claimed, but it is also essential to inform the strategic formulation of health policies, and for the monitoring and evaluation of interventions designed to reduce inequalities and improve overall population health. These are among the fundamental goals of any health system, yet there is very little evidence that health systems are responding appropriately to the changes in disease patterns that are occurring throughout much of the developing world. If the meta-synthesis of data and information offered by the ongoing Global Burden of Disease Study is any indication, we are witnessing a rapid disease transition from conditions that mostly affect the health and survival of mothers and children to conditions that primarily affect young and middle-aged adults. Yet health systems, donor priorities, and the structural orientation of the World Health Organization are changing too slowly, if at all, to this new and rapidly evolving global epidemiological environment.

In an era of limited resources for health, it is important that these are allocated most rationally to improve the overall health of the population, and particularly that of the least well off. There is convincing evidence that the global response to reducing maternal and child deaths is working: the annual number of child deaths has halved since 1990 and is likely to halve again by 2030. However, health policies and health systems are not adapting rapidly enough to this success of having many more children surviving to adolescence. Surely the goal of all societies must be to not only keep babies alive until adolescence, but adolescents alive to old age as well. If that is a universally acceptable moral commitment to which a modern society should aspire, then how well prepared are we to do so?

Appallingly badly it would seem. The focus of global health efforts over the past half century on improving child survival has not been accompanied by comparable interest in reducing the leading causes of death in young and middle-aged adults. The single exception is HIV/AIDS which still kills around 1 million young adults each year. But what kills the other 12 million people who die every year between the ages of 15 and 60? If we are to take mortality reduction in this age group seriously, we need to better understand the other leading causes of death at these ages. We need to know which causes result in greatest loss of potential life, and where and in which population subgroups they are most rampant. We need to understand how the composition of leading causes of death is changing, and the principal risk factors that underlie these epidemiological patterns. Collectively, this data will inform national debates about priority interventions to reduce adult mortality, and to evaluate how successful they have been in preventing premature death. Yet the massive data assessment effort that characterizes the Global Burden of Disease Study has confirmed that very few low- and middle-income countries have functioning cause-of-death systems. In those countries where deaths are registered, the accuracy of the cause-of-death assignment is very poor, greatly limiting the policy value of the data. Indeed, the deplorable state of vital registration systems worldwide means that cause-of-death patterns in countries can only be estimated with vast and unacceptable uncertainty.

How can we access critical information on cause of death that is sufficiently timely and accurate so that it's useful? Medical certification of all deaths is unlikely to be widespread nor affordable in most developing countries in our lifetime. Moreover, research has repeatedly identified systematic misclassification of the cause of death of those who die in hospitals in developing countries, greatly reducing the value of this information to guide national health planning. While a systematic, concerted, and strategic effort by countries to improve the accuracy of hospital-certified causes of death is a priority, so too is the application of recent advances in "verbal autopsy" methods that can cost-effectively measure causes of death using automated computer algorithms that recognize and associate response patterns more reliably than physicians can. Moreover, these methods are cheap, quick, readily implemented, and do not take physicians away from their essential clinical care duties.

Global leadership and support is urgently needed to introduce new cause-of-death methods in developing countries in parallel with the establishment of sample death registration systems. This could rapidly and cheaply improve the evidence base about leading causes of death among adults and provide essential information to guide policies designed to ensure their survival into old age.

Alan Lopez is a Melbourne Laureate Professor and the Rowden-White Chair of Global Health and Burden of Disease Measurement at the University of Melbourne.

Chapter 60

Five Pillars of Wisdom

ADETOKUNBO O. LUCAS

The past, present, and future of global health rests on five pillars: ethics, research, management, partnerships, and goals.

The past few decades have witnessed remarkable advances in addressing health issues on a global plane. These creative and intensified programs are usually described under the general term *global health*. The term is widely used in discussing international health programs, in naming and renaming institutions and their departments, and in labeling academic undertakings that reflect modern concepts on health issues.

As often happens to such widely used terms, there is no clear consensus as to the exact definition of global health. A useful approach would be to identify and collate the characteristic features of global health and define the term on the basis of its essential features.

On the basis of lessons learned, the essential features of global health can be summarized under five headings: (1) a sound ethical foundation; (2) health research; (3) the strategic design and management of health programs; (4) partnerships; and (5) global goals and targets.

A sound ethical foundation of equity and social justice is fundamental to global health. One of the most important contributions of the public health discipline has been drawing attention to the economic and social factors that affect health. Studies by statisticians and demographers have produced convincing evidence of the deleterious effect of poverty on human health. The adage "the poor die young" draws attention to the vicious cycle linking poverty to disease, disability, and premature death. Public health workers have been at the forefront of advocating for economic and social interventions in packages aimed at improving health.

Health research is an essential component of the global health package. It calls for a comprehensive approach that is inclusive of insights and methods from multiple disciplines including biomedical, social, and economics studies. Ultimately, the goal is to ensure that all health decisions are rooted in knowledge and science. This means global health's research agenda must cover assessments of the distributions and dimensions of health and disease; analysis of health systems; development of new and improved technologies for disease control; and basic research in human biology and related environmental factors.

The strategic design and management of health programs is needed to ensure that they are efficient, effective, cost-effective, and equitable. To achieve these goals, health workers have designed and tested creative and innovative approaches. A recent example of a successful innovation is community-directed intervention with ivermectin, an antiparasitic medicine; this approach has found useful application for other mass treatment programs. Monitoring and evaluation of global health projects is also important. This provides useful information about need, demand for services, input of services, outputs, outcomes, and impact.

Partnerships involving collaborative ventures are essential features of global health programs. Ideally, such collaboration includes all relevant stakeholders: the public and private sectors; for-profit and nonprofit actors; developed and developing countries; and so on. The essence of such partnerships is a collective goal, joint investment of resources and expertise, and a fair sharing of outputs. The reciprocal relationship among partners generates mutual benefits for all the participants.

Global goals and targets like the Millennium Development Goals have encouraged national governments around the world to improve the health of pregnant women, children, and other vulnerable groups. Other actions included the intensified control of HIV/AIDS, malaria, tuberculosis, and other major infectious diseases. Additionally, medical interventions have been complemented with economic and social interventions aimed at reducing poverty.

The eradication of smallpox is an illustrative example of the value of global health programs when these five pillars come together. The old-fashioned approach by which each country strives to protect its population against cross-border transmission of epidemic diseases does little or nothing in eradicating the disease. The global eradication of smallpox was finally achieved only through a coordinated global effort. The global health approach can be effectively applied for the control of cancers, cardiovascular diseases, and other noncommunicable diseases.

To conclude, in the coming decades, the global health community will continue its struggle against the unfinished business of persisting infectious diseases like HIV/AIDS, tuberculosis, and malaria. In most communities, priorities will shift increasingly toward the growing problems that noncommunicable diseases pose. One can, with cautious optimism, hope that global health—as defined by the five pillars of wisdom—will lead to brilliant achievements. As we move forward, these five pillars should be used as a checklist for the performance of global health.

Adetokunbo O. Lucas is an Adjunct Professor of Global Health and Population at the Harvard T.H. Chan School of Public Health and former Director of the World Health Organization's Tropical Diseases Research Programme.

Chapter 61

Keeping the Promise to Children

GRAÇA MACHEL

Child health has come a long way in the last two decades; maintaining that trajectory is the next step.

Most people are not aware that in the space of a generation, the rate at which children are dying has been cut in half. In 1990, close to 1 in 10 children died before their fifth birthday, and in some countries, this number was closer to 1 in 5. By 2013, the number of children dying before age 5 had fallen from 90 deaths per 1,000 births to 46, and this number continues to fall. Over the past 22 years, the world has saved around 90 million lives that might have otherwise been lost had mortality rates remained at the 1990 levels. That's more than the entire population of Germany.

This is an amazing trend, perhaps the most important trend in global health today. The increased availability and affordability of lifesaving interventions has played a major part in this trend. This includes the focus on the first 1,000 days of life, immunization, vitamin A, insecticide-treated bed nets, and community-based management of acute malnutrition.

But what has really catalyzed this transformation has been the commitment and engagement that we have seen from governments and communities worldwide. Today, the countries with the highest rates of child mortality are stepping up efforts to accelerate declines and build on the momentum we've seen over the past 25 years. For example, in 2012, the governments of Ethiopia, India, and the United States—together with UNICEF—brought together more than 700 partners from the public, private, and civil society sectors for the Child Survival Call to Action. This resulted in a rejuvenated global movement for child survival, *Committing to Child Survival: A Promise Renewed,* and since then, 178 governments have signed a pledge vowing to redouble efforts to accelerate declines in child mortality.

But while commitment is strong and progress has been incredible, 46 deaths for every 1,000 births still equates to 6.3 million children who die every year, denied the chance to grow up and live full, meaningful lives. And while the number of deaths continues to fall, serious challenges that stand in our way are slowing progress.

Rates of newborn mortality are not falling as fast as they should. Nearly half of all under age 5 deaths now occur during the first 28 days, with 2.8 million children dying before their 28th day of life. Every year, one million children die on their birthday—their first and only day of life. What makes this even more unacceptable is the fact that most of these deaths could be prevented by simple, affordable interventions. Research has given us the evidence and causes of these problems, so there is no excuse why these lives cannot be saved. By focusing greater energy on this newborn period and these simple interventions, we can achieve huge gains quickly.

We must work to improve equity, both at the global level and within countries. The most recent data show that West and Central Africa continues to shoulder the world's largest burden of child mortality, with one in eight children dying before the age of 5. In many countries, coverage of lifesaving services is unacceptably low among the poorest and most marginalised. We must address these global injustices and make certain that no mother, no child, is left behind.

This is the reason why I am engaged with *Committing to Child Survival: A Promise Renewed,* the global effort to stop all children from dying of causes that are easily prevented. Under the banner of this movement, governments are translating promises into action—by sharpening national strategies and setting bold, new targets for maternal, newborn, and child survival.

I am absolutely convinced that when we invest in women and children, we invest in transformative change. As a woman, a mother, and a grandmother watching the next generations grow, struggle, and thrive, I feel a deep responsibility to take action. I stand committed to improving the lives of my continent's youngest and most vulnerable citizens. Please, join me. Together, we can ignite an African movement and bring about a renaissance for maternal and child survival.

Graça Machel is Founder of the Graça Machel Trust, Chair of the World Health Organization's Partnership for Maternal, Newborn, and Child Health, Chancellor of the University of Cape Town, former First Lady of Mozambique and South Africa, and former Chair of Gavi, the Vaccine Alliance.

Chapter 62

Embracing Community Innovation

MATHURA MAHENDREN

We must move beyond community acceptance and push for community innovation, where local ideas are not only elicited, but they are integral to the development of innovations for health and health care.

As we head into what promises to be a revolutionary period for global development and innovation, we must redefine the role of the community in the consultative process. It will no longer be enough to aim for community acceptance and support of initiatives. We must instead push for community innovation, where local ideas are not only elicited, but are integral in the development of innovations for health and health care.

During my undergraduate studies, I had the privilege of working with a grassroots NGO in Mzuzu, Malawi. One day when visiting an eco-sanitation project in a nearby village named Ekayiweni, we observed that while the new eco-toilets were well-received by the community, the accompanying handwashing stations—bottles suspended from two sticks—were not. At almost 80% of the stations, the bottles were empty, and the ground beneath was completely dry. Despite being briefed on the importance of such sanitary procedures in preventing disease, the villagers did not see the value in handwashing. It left me frustrated. Why didn't they understand? Furthermore, this was a community-based solution, and by the books, it should work. So why wasn't it?

An answer came in the form of an elderly woman who had planted a sweet potato garden directly beneath her handwashing station so that the water would also be supporting her crop. Not only was she making efficient use of all-available resources, but now she had extra incentive to wash her hands. This inspiring innovator made me realize how much community *innovation*—not just consultation or engagement—matters in implementing development initiatives. My peers and I had assumed that awareness would be incentive enough, and in trying repeatedly to instill community members with the importance of handwashing for their health, we had lost sight of potential alternatives. Her solution made so much sense, yet this was an idea that neither myself nor any of my peers would have formulated on our own. She was an example of the undiscovered and unharnessed expertise that lies within a community itself, and through her actions alone, she taught me to listen before I speak, to observe before I act, to ask before I assume.

By asking, I learned that the eco-sanitation project was designed by researchers at the local Mzuzu University. While there were community conversations that happened beforehand to gauge local interest in the project, and follow-up conversations to ensure that the program was doing well, there were no explicit calls for innovation from the community.

To harness community expertise, we need to admit to ourselves something that appears to be so difficult for so many of us to do: that is, to say, "I don't know." Then we must understand that there may be others who do know, that may have the knowledge that we don't, and that they may not have multiple letters after their names. We need to acknowledge this fact in our work globally and at home.

It is not enough to have the community sign off on an initiative after the fact. We need to include and engage communities in the process of innovation, and value their insights as insider perspectives. Only then can we ensure that initiatives withstand the test of time, resources, and local beliefs. Furthermore, innovations that emerge from within communities are likely to be more cost-effective and sustainable as they are built using locally available resources.

For those working in the innovation sector, scaling-up is always a concern. As I promote community innovation, I must at the same time mention that these innovations cannot be replicated, packaged, and airdropped into neighboring communities or countries as originally conceived. While the learning from local initiatives should always be shared, each community is different and will require adaptations or innovations to suit its unique context and needs.

So what can we do?

At the systems level, we must advocate for processes that incentivize the prioritization of community innovation. Depending on the system, this may mean tying funding for research and development to community involvement in project design, mandating that communities have increased representation in bodies that govern which ideas are implemented, and encouraging local experts to take the lead in implementing initiatives on the ground.

As individuals, we can start by asking a few more questions. Instead of stopping with "Do you support the implementation of this project in your community?" or "Do you believe you will benefit from this effort?", we must ask "How do you think we can improve this design?" or "Is there anything you think we should change?" These are simple questions, but I think we'll be surprised by the responses we receive—just as I was surprised by the elder innovator I met in Ekayiweni.

Let us remember that if global health is our final destination, then community innovation must be our trusted compass.

Mathura Mahendren is a BHSc (Honours) candidate at McMaster University and former intern with Ungweru in Mzuzu, Malawi.

Chapter 63

Fairness and Health Equity

MICHAEL MARMOT

If social injustice is to be addressed once and for all, we need to put health equity at the heart of all policymaking, globally and nationally.

Here are two difficult questions. First, what constitutes a just society? Philosopher Stuart Hampshire argues that there is no one answer to this question. Libertarians may give priority to equality of rights, Rawlsians to equality of initial conditions, and Amartya Sen to equality of capabilities. The kind of society to which these three different approaches might give rise would look quite different. I have an answer: the just society is one that gives rise to health equity, where health inequity is defined as those systematic inequalities in health between social groups that are avoidable by reasonable means.

Second question: in the face of the kind of financial shock of 2008 that led to the Great Recession, what is the appropriate policy response? In Europe, the Troika of the European Commission, International Monetary Fund, and European Central Bank imposed severe policies of austerity on "wayward" European countries. It was believed that countries with high national debts and high budget deficits could only return to economic growth by cutting their deficits. Opponents of this approach argued that investing in the economy was the way forward, and believed that economic growth was necessary in reducing deficits. Once again, these two views lead to radically different policies: the former to reduction in public spending, the latter to increases. Which is right? Economists disagree. My answer is of the same form that I give to the philosophers: the right macroeconomic policy is one that favors health equity.

Underlying my answer to both of these questions is a judgment and a claim. The judgement is that the way society is organized has profound effects on the lives people are able to lead, their health, and the fair distribution of health, or health equity. The claim is that we should organize society on moral principles. A "fair" distribution of health—health equity—is a moral principle. Such an approach is in sharp contrast to our present way of doing things nationally and globally. Today, most societies and international negotiations are organized on the basis of inequities in power, money, and resources. In fact, "social injustice is killing on a grand scale" was the way the World Health Organization's Commission on Social Determinants of Health summarized the current state of affairs globally.

Thomas Piketty, a French economist, captured worldwide interest with his prediction that, in the twenty-first century, rich countries are heading toward the kind of inequalities in wealth last seen in the nineteenth century. We are busily recreating patrimonial capitalism where vast wealth continues to grow faster than do incomes, and this inequity is passed on to succeeding generations. As a result, "rewards" are distributed according to rent and privilege. There are many reasons why this is not a desirable state of affairs, not least that it conflicts with the democratic ideal that effort and merit, let alone need, are fairer ways of distributing economic reward. However, the most important reason for concern with inequities in income and wealth distribution, within and between countries, is their impact on health and health equity.

In making this connection, I understand that by placing health equity at the heart of all policymaking we would be organizing our societies and our global community in a way that is fundamentally different from those organized on the basis of powerful special interests and some version of market fundamentalism. As such, we must put into practice the good evidence that has been gathered on social determinants of health through the life course—early child development, education, employment and working conditions, and healthy and sustainable houses and communities—thereby guaranteeing that everyone in society has the minimum income necessary to lead a life of dignity. At the center of these practical policies is empowering individuals and communities to have control over their lives.

Michael Marmot is Professor of Epidemiology and Public Health and Director of the Institute of Health Equity at University College London; President-Elect of the World Medical Association; and former Chair of the World Health Organization's Commission on Social Determinants of Health.

Chapter 64

Medicines Must Be Safer

MALEBONA PRECIOUS MATSOSO

We must improve how medicines are regulated because everyone is hurt by unnecessary adverse drug reactions.

Medical product injuries are a big problem. While medicines are designed to heal, too often they cause unnecessary harm, hospitalization, and death. These injuries are a significant burden to public health and a challenge for new drug development. Just like diseases that know no boundaries, these medicines are distributed across countries and consumed worldwide. It is our responsibility to work globally to ensure that medical products are made safer for all.

I have witnessed firsthand the devastating effects of unsafe medicines. Toxic Epidermal Necrolysis (TEN) and its milder counterpart Steven John Syndrome (SJS) are both potentially fatal skin diseases that are most often caused by adverse drug reactions.

My first encounter with an SJS case was a painful one. Sophie, a patient in my hospital, was unrecognizable, with completely shut and swollen eyes, and blisters covering her whole body and mouth. She unfortunately died. To date, more than 200 medications, including antibiotics, antiretrovirals, and anticonvulsants, have been reported to be associated with SJS/TEN. Many of them are still prescribed. Incidence and severity of these reactions are greater in those with HIV/AIDS and other infections. While these drugs may save many from the potentially debilitating effects of some diseases, it is equally important to ensure that people are spared the pain and agony of the adverse reactions these medicines often cause.

Before a new prescription medicine is put on the market, it must first be approved for sale by a medicine regulatory authority. In South Africa, this is the Medicines Control Council. In the United States, it's the Food and Drug Administration. Approval of medicines is always based on three criteria: quality, efficacy, and safety. Unnecessary risks can be avoided by ensuring that these regulatory bodies base their approval decisions on thorough risk–benefit analyses. Furthermore, once medicines are widely available, they must be constantly monitored for safety and quality, and withdrawn immediately should they present unexpected health risks or severe adverse effects.

It takes only three simple facts to realize the immensity of this problem.

First, regulatory system failures represent unnecessary costs—to patients in loss of life, to industry in loss of revenue through litigation costs, and to society as a whole in loss of health and well-being. The public is ultimately on the receiving end of unsafe products that contribute to harm, so we all have a stake in improving this situation.

Second, unsafe products deplete limited health-care resources that are desperately needed elsewhere. Health Ministries just don't have enough money to waste any. Projected hospitalization costs to the British National Health Service associated with adverse drug reactions are about $847 million USD per year. A recent study in South Africa estimated that adverse drug reactions cost 483,000 ZAR for just two of my country's many medical wards. This extrapolates to 1.9 million ZAR that cannot be spent on effective interventions. There are also payouts for court claims and legal fees.

Third, those who have been harmed by unsafe medical products deserve meaningful compensation, and too often victims receive a small fraction of the payouts or none at all. In addition to monetary compensation, accountability requires addressing the industry and regulatory failures that enabled the injury in the first place. Only then can we bring about restoration.

As a first step to addressing the safety problem, we must introduce preventative measures to avoid adverse drug reactions. This means that harmful products should be withdrawn globally based on universal standards. Since 1979, the United Nations General Assembly has compiled a list of banned pharmaceutical products. Over a period of four decades, that list has grown in size and scope of application. Today it includes over 1,100 products regulated in 115 countries. Unfortunately, its implementation has been less satisfactory, with no firm commitment by countries. Adverse drug reactions can only be prevented if we take a firm global stance against unsafe medical products and hold countries accountable for their regulatory decisions.

Prevention also requires reducing the excessive consumption of drugs that is driven by pharmaceutical companies pursuing illegal marketing strategies and misleading consumers, such as when they promote unapproved and untested uses of their products that were cleared only for particular diseases and conditions. The world's top ten pharmaceutical firms spent $739 billion USD globally from 1996 to 2005 on marketing and administration. A significant amount is also spent on promotional samples that are distributed free to patients. To stop such crazy levels of expenditure, we must start levying industry on their marketing costs and use this revenue to fund public education on the appropriate use of medicines.

Ultimately, governments around the world must work without delay to reduce socially adverse behavior by the pharmaceutical industry and promote conduct that is safety enhancing. Global debates thus far have not focused on medical product safety. Let the world show it cares about the public's health by making medicines safer. So much can be achieved if only we work together.

Malebona Precious Matsoso is the Director-General of the South African Department of Health and former Director of Public Health, Innovation, and Intellectual Property for the World Health Organization.

Chapter 65

From Hegemony to Partnership

ANNE MILLS

Changing health needs, growing demands for health care, and increased resources demand new ways of working together that reflect genuine partnership across countries.

In recent decades there has been a considerable increase in development assistance for health, and a proliferation of global funding agencies and initiatives focused on specific diseases or health problems. While development assistance has provided funding to address major causes of ill-health, it has also resulted in multiple, often poorly coordinated, programs and projects.

There is a long history of attempts to reshape the aid architecture, including agreements such as the Paris Declaration on Aid Effectiveness and the Accra Agenda for Action, which emphasize country ownership, donor alignment with country strategies, and harmonization of donor actions. Yet, despite promising initiatives like the International Health Partnership, the agendas of agencies in the rich world—governments, civil society groups, industry—still dominate the global health arena. At regular intervals a new lobby develops to promote their pet disease or problem, often via a new institutional mechanism. This is not to say that HIV/AIDS, malaria, neglected tropical diseases, or maternal and child health are unimportant. Rather, it is concerning that their rise to prominence reflects internal dynamics within and between high-income countries rather than open debates and discussions with recipient countries.

The health sector seems especially prone to this hegemony—one might hypothesize because of the specialized nature of the medical profession and the existence of strong advocates for particular diseases, technologies such as vaccination, or population groups.

The pursuit of specific initiatives has an especially pernicious effect on the development of country health systems. Multiple initiatives fragment sources of support to the health sector, duplicate core systems such as drug procurement, compete for the best health workers, and overstress limited management capacity. While offers of substantial funds for good causes are hard for recipient countries to refuse, they create advocacy groups within countries themselves, making coherent local policy more difficult to achieve.

In the rich world, health system issues such as financing sources, organizational structures, and quality of care dominate health debates. The debate on services for specific diseases or population groups occurs within the context of the overall system and how the system manages these diseases or groups. Why then is it so difficult to conceptualize and structure our engagement on health with poorer countries in this way?

During my involvement with the first Copenhagen Consensus process—which examined how best to invest in solving global problems based on cost–benefit criteria—the reaction of two different interest groups to my analyses of the costs and benefits of control of HIV/AIDS, malaria control, and scaled-up basic health services was illuminating. Whereas a panel of world-leading economists ranked control of HIV/AIDS first of all problems across all sectors, given its very favorable benefit–cost ratio, a panel of UN ambassadors and senior diplomats from 24 countries, including 16 low- and middle-income countries, ranked scaled-up basic health services first despite the somewhat lower benefit–cost ratio. I remember their justification very clearly: how can a country sustain disease control without broader health system support? Why focus on just one disease when people who visit health facilities often need care for unclear or multiple conditions?

In the coming decades, political and economic relationships between current aid donors and recipient countries will be dramatically changed, especially given rapid economic transformations in many African and Asian countries. National health systems will be even more exposed to global influences, in the form of transnational medical, pharmaceutical, and health-care industries, movement of health workers, expectations of services given knowledge of people's levels of access to health care in other countries, or widely disseminated information from global benchmarking of the performance of national health systems. Current low- and middle-income countries will face critical questions of how best to shape the development of their health systems given changing health needs, growing demands for health care, and increased resources. Exchange between countries will become less based on financial transfers, and more on sharing of experiences and technical advice based on evidence of what works in various country contexts.

To address these health and system challenges, which increasingly transcend national boundaries, we must rapidly evolve new ways of working across the world that reflect genuine partnership and lesson-learning across countries.

Anne Mills is Deputy Director, Provost, and Professor of Health Economics and Policy with the London School of Hygiene and Tropical Medicine, and former President of the International Health Economics Association.

Chapter 66

Health in the Global Economy

SUERIE MOON

We need to place greater value on health in global rulemaking to move toward a more sustainable global society.

The health of a population is a central indicator of the health of a society. "The first wealth," Ralph Waldo Emerson said, "is health." While health has consistently been ranked among the highest values across societies and across time, we continue to live in an era in which economic goals, policies, and indicators nearly always take precedence. Globalization has created not only economic interdependence, but also health interdependence, such that not even the most powerful countries can protect the health of their populations by acting alone. Yet the rules that we have constructed thus far to govern globalization tend to privilege economic concerns, with inadequate consideration given to health.

For example, cross-border investment flows are currently governed by a web of over 3,000 investment treaties that foreign firms can use to restrict national public health legislation, in addition to other laws affecting important social determinants of health, such as labor and environmental regulations. Recently, the tobacco firm Philip Morris used such treaties to mount legal challenges to tobacco control laws in Uruguay and Australia. In addition, intellectual property rules contained in multilateral and bilateral trade agreements have markedly strengthened and lengthened monopoly protection on medicines in developing countries, enabling higher prices for longer periods of time.

Finally, many internationally backed austerity measures intended to counteract the global economic crisis that began in 2008 focused on restarting economic growth, with insufficient attention to simultaneously protecting public health.

The problem is not only that global economic rules can undermine public health, but also that such rules tend to be stronger, more formalized, and backed by enforcement mechanisms. In contrast, with a few important exceptions such as the Framework Convention on Tobacco Control or the International Health Regulations, global rules for health tend to be weaker, less formal, with little or no means to ensure compliance. The problem is not the absence of international normative standards for health, such as codes of conduct negotiated to regulate the marketing of breast milk substitute, the international recruitment of health workers, or marketing of alcohol to minors. Binding economic agreements do sometimes contain health exceptions that should be exploited far more frequently than they are. Key examples are the public health safeguards in the World Trade Organization's intellectual property agreement. But normative exhortations and health exceptions are a poor substitute for the purposeful negotiation of strong global rules for public health, especially in an era of increasing health interdependence. A sobering reminder of this problem is the recent attempt to launch negotiations on a binding global treaty to finance research and development for medicines needed by populations in developing countries, which fell flat when governments were collectively unwilling to make binding commitments.

So what is it that we need for global health? We need stronger global rulemaking to manage the situation of health interdependence that characterizes the world today. Such rulemaking needs to both promote effective cross-border regulations with the intention of protecting health, and ensure that health is adequately protected in rulemaking that takes place in the economic sphere.

However, currently we lack both the institutional arrangements and the normative basis in society to get there. The institution mandated with convening states to negotiate global norms and rules for health—the World Health Organization—is poorly equipped to do so because, in part, of its inadequate financing structure. This weakness has its roots at the national level, where the conventional wisdom is that ministries of health are and will always be weaker than ministries of foreign affairs, trade, or finance. In other words, policymakers collectively privilege economy over health. Ironically, they continue to do so despite the growing realization that health and wealth are intrinsically interconnected and can mutually reinforce or undermine each other.

In the long run, we need broader normative shifts in society that put as great a value on health in policymaking as individual citizens do. Changes in infant mortality, life expectancy, and health disparities in a society should share the front pages with changes in economic growth rates, GDP, and unemployment. At the same time, we need enlightened political leadership, both within and outside the health sector, which values and forcefully asserts health concerns in global economic rulemaking. Such changes in societal values, policymaking, and leadership are essential if we are to move toward a more sustainable global society.

Suerie Moon is Co-Chair of the Forum on Global Governance for Health at the Harvard Global Health Institute and a Lecturer in the Department of Global Health and Population at the Harvard T.H. Chan School of Public Health.

Chapter 67

Disability and a Healthy Society

CHAELI MYCROFT

Disability is a universal health issue; now it needs to be seen as a social and equality issue too.

Disability is a global issue and people with disabilities form a significant part of the world's population. Yet, as one of the largest minorities, the rights of people with disabilities are often the rights that are the least advocated for. As a result, their voices often go unheard. This is problematic if our aim is to have a healthy, inclusive society.

Disability is more than just a health issue; it is a social issue that cuts across and impacts all spheres of life. This is not only true for people living with disabilities but also for their families, their friends, and their communities. Everybody in society is affected by disability in some way, be it directly or indirectly. Disability is quite an interesting challenge in and of itself, because it is entirely possible for any person to acquire an impairment in his or her lifetime—through developing health problems or through an accident—and this creates an intriguing attitude toward disability that needs unpacking.

Living with a mobility impairment myself, I feel I can comment on the challenges of physical accessibility—a very real barrier in my everyday life. Our environment disempowers people when they are unable to enter a building independently because the infrastructure of buildings and surrounding terrain do not allow this to happen. However, when we are faced with disempowering environments we can choose to be discouraged, or we can choose to empower ourselves and educate others about these challenges. More open discourse is needed, and we must all actively advocate for our right to physically access our world.

In my experience, every disability issue under discussion often leads to the same underlying problem, with many challenges arising as a result of financial difficulty. Being disabled is expensive. Regardless of what impairment a person may have, that person has special needs that require financial support. Assistive devices cost huge amounts of money and many people with disabilities come from poorer backgrounds, especially in my country, South Africa. This makes it exceptionally difficult to integrate people with disabilities into mainstream society. Transport is a significant barrier and the cost of servicing assistive devices and providing for interventions in the form of various therapies speak to the financial constraints created by living with a mobility impairment. In many cases the products on which people with disabilities rely for general living are provided by very few service providers—often creating a monopoly which results in high prices.

We cannot simply consider disability as an issue to be dealt with by those who experience it directly. We need to work together as a global community to create a society where each member is acknowledged for his or her potential strengths instead of potential weaknesses. In that way we can heal society and make it an inclusive and positive place for all.

Chaeli Mycroft is a Co-Founder of The Chaeli Campaign and winner of the 2011 Children's Peace Prize, 2012 Nobel Peace Laureates' Medal for Social Activism, and 2013 World of Children Youth Award.

Chapter 68

Fusion Fund for Health

SANIA NISHTAR

By combining grants and loans into fusion funds, we can create an innovative solution for the millions of people suffering from the consequences of catastrophic health expenditures.

Four cases epitomize a problem that millions face worldwide: either the family is at the brink of medically ushered financial catastrophe or the patient risks forgoing health care.

A four-year-old girl with a correctable congenital heart defect will surely die without treatment; her parents are in the process of borrowing money from informal moneylenders, who charge usurious rates on loans.

A 70-year-old woman, who was taken away from the hospital with a broken hip is bedridden for life because her family cannot afford the operation.

A daily-wage laborer with cancer, the only breadwinner in a poor family of 17, cannot afford treatment even after selling two goats, his only source of livelihood.

A relatively well-to-do woman with renal failure is undergoing fortnightly dialysis, while her family has sold most household assets to keep her alive.

More than 250 million people suffer similar consequences worldwide and a quarter of the world's population, living below the poverty line, are at risk of medical impoverishment, debt, or foregoing treatment when faced with high-cost health care. But this problem is not limited to the poor: catastrophic health expenditures are pervasive in all settings where people pay out-of-pocket for health care. Even in developed countries like the United States, financial barriers to health care often exist—even for the insured.

Health insurance is considered the primary tool against health-related financial calamity in many health systems. However, insurance may not provide full coverage against catastrophic costs. Explicit entitlements in some other health systems, where health care is meant to be provided free at point of service, also usually do not cover high-cost expenditures.

This calls for innovations, which can be seen as additional financing approaches, to achieve universal health coverage.

Current solutions to address catastrophic health expenditures are fragmented. Developing countries grapple with social health insurance as a tool, with only a few examples of health equity funds that actually work to overcome financial barriers for the poor. Some microfinance institutions have piloted health loans as a second-generation product to help the poor break the cycle of ill health and poverty. In emerging market countries, non-banking financial institutions and the corporate sector have experimented with providing consumer loans to patients with health-care needs. In the United States, "zero-interest" and high-interest health loans are available, both for one-time catastrophic costs as well as for bridging gaps in health insurance. Catastrophic insurance plans, with high deductibles, albeit with entitlement to a tax-advantaged medical savings account, are an additional option.

Most of these "solutions" are problematic. Social health insurance with premiums that governments can underwrite do not cover catastrophic costs, and grant-based health equity funds are unsustainable. Health savings accounts may not pay high-cost deductibles. Health loans come with inherent risks since they do not correspond with an income-generating action and are accordingly plagued by the moral hazard of "refusals on the grounds of lack of creditworthiness." Other financing plans entertain only the creditworthy.

These problems can be overcome with a fusion fund where a medical loan program can be combined with a grant window. The creditworthy can be served from the loan window and others can be considered for grants. A third component, a "support window," could underwrite bad loans, subsidize interest, and allow reasonable grace periods in repayment.

In a three-window fusion fund, the risk of one financing approach can be offset with another. The moral hazard of "refusals" in health loans can be offset through the grant window. The grant side could be made sustainable by ploughing the profits of the loan's operation and through investments. Access to these financing options can be tied to the applicant's socioeconomic condition. Tools exist to enable ascertainment of patients' eligibility and, hence, applicants can be triaged to either window.

In setting up a fusion fund, operational lessons from pilot health loan programs and grant-making funds, which provide assistance to protect the poor against catastrophic expenditure, can be instructive. Several innovations employing the use of technology, mobile phones, and crowdsourcing approaches have been tested to improve targeting and transparency. These experiences can inform fund utilization.

Beyond serving as a safety net for the poor, a fusion fund would also be a financing instrument to protect the non-poor against catastrophic expenditures on health. It can be structured as a sustainable proposition while also having a social mission. Such an instrument could potentially be a replacement for individual financial coping strategies, which lead to catastrophic costs, impoverishment, bankruptcies, and foregone care.

Sania Nishtar is the Founder of Heartfile and the former Pakistani Federal Minister for Science and Technology, Education and Trainings, and Information Technology and Telcom, with additional responsibility for Health.

Chapter 69

Health and Not Health Care

ANDERS NORDSTRÖM

We must shift the global health paradigm from disease to health, from survival to staying healthy, and from health care to health as a key dimension of development.

To tackle present and future global health challenges we need a paradigm shift. Our perspectives and strategies must move upstream—from merely providing health services to ensuring that people both survive and remain healthy throughout the course of their lives. Improving access to vaccines and increasing prevention and treatment of disease will not be enough to realize this vision for a healthy future.

The focus must be on creating healthier societies. There are critical opportunities to engage and stimulate other sectors—agriculture, food production, infrastructure, urban planning, and energy production—to not only achieve their sector-specific objectives, but to contribute substantially to better health. The door is open for these win-win deals. Top priorities in undertaking these partnerships should be facilitating access to more nutritious foods, increasing levels of physical activity, and reducing smoking and alcohol intake. Junk food and soft drinks should not be allowed in schools or associated with sports activities. It should be easier to take the stairs instead of the elevator, and the bike instead of the car.

Simply put, what is good for our planet is good for people's health, and what is good for health is good for sustainable development.

It is also time to engage in a proactive but differentiated dialogue with the private sector, with the exception of the tobacco industry for which such engagement is unwarranted. The production of alcohol and beverages we have to accept, but reducing people's consumption is critical. The food industry is different and here to stay. However, through a combination of regulations, price incentives, and consumer power, the food available needs to become radically healthier. Antibiotics in our meat need to go, the amount of sugar in processed foods must be dramatically reduced, and trans fats should be abandoned altogether.

The health system needs to become a system where health care is provided but where promotion and prevention are just as important. The health system has to be more explicit about its role in advising and influencing other sectors, including transportation and infrastructure.

Is the current global health system fit for such a different agenda and approach? Do we have the right dialogue and partnerships between public and private actors to effect this change? Are people empowered and equipped to make healthier choices for their lives? No, probably not.

To respond to the future health agenda, the global system needs to cater to the production of global public goods, such as research and knowledge, innovation and technologies, as well as global agreements or potentially legally binding conventions. Creating healthier societies and providing opportunities for people to make healthy choices does not necessarily require additional financial resources, but it does call for a change in policies and behaviors.

Leadership from the World Health Organization is crucial in this effort and must be more ambitious in terms of multi-sectorial action and engagement. The alternative would be to build on the HIV/AIDS experience and transform the Joint United Nations Program on HIV/AIDS into a UNHEALTH or to ask the United Nations Development Program to take on health as a development issue. I would not favor that.

The bottom line is that we need to think of health instead of health care. This will require a major shift in mindset, resource allocation, and political priorities.

Anders Nordström is Sweden's Ambassador for Global Health and former Acting Director-General of the World Health Organization.

Chapter 70

Diet for a Healthy Future

NGOZI OKONJO-IWEALA

Changing dietary and lifestyle patterns emanating from a rising middle class represents a massive health and development risk that requires urgent attention.

Significant economic growth in developing countries has lifted millions out of poverty and created a new middle class. Countries like China and India have recorded annual economic growth rates as high as 9% over the last decade. Africa is also part of this growth trend as host to six of the ten fastest growing economies. With economic growth, millions of households in developing countries have been lifted out of poverty and into middle-class status. In Africa, between 1980 and 2010, the middle class rose from about 126 million (27% of the population) to 350 million people (34% of the population).

This increase in the number of middle-class households around the world is leading to dramatic changes in dietary patterns, including greater demand for meat and dairy products. In addition, lifestyles are becoming more sedentary as more formal jobs are created.

Such dietary and lifestyle changes resulting from economic growth have adverse health consequences. Diets heavy on meats, fats, and carbohydrates contribute to the development of noncommunicable diseases like obesity, diabetes, high blood pressure, and cancer, all of which are currently exploding in developing countries. On a personal note, given the amount of daily stress in my job and especially as I get older,

I have had to reorient my own diet and lifestyle to ensure continued good health. More fish, smaller helpings of carbohydrates, and exercise four times a week appears to be working. The negative health consequences of dietary changes are compounded where increased alcohol and tobacco intake accompany these changing dietary patterns. In the past five years, over $600 million USD has been invested by alcohol and tobacco production companies in Nigeria alone, according to government statistics.

Unfortunately, health systems of most developing countries are far from able to cope with this increase in noncommunicable diseases on top of the disproportionate burden they already face. Indeed, nearly 80% of NCD deaths from noncommunicable diseases occur in developing countries. The World Health Organization projects that by 2020 the largest increases in noncommunicable disease deaths will occur in Africa. This grim picture partly reflects the serious weaknesses in African health systems. Treating most noncommunicable diseases is expensive, complex, and requires highly skilled health workers, who are absent in many African countries. With health expenditures that are largely private and out-of-pocket, this will undoubtedly have significant impact on household finances and the health of the overall economy.

The solution is as technical as it is socioeconomic. Our orientation should be toward more cost-effective prevention strategies rather than more expensive curative services. We must educate a new class of consumers, and reorient lifestyles and dietary patterns in a healthier direction through effective health promotion. The availability of fitness centers in schools and at the workplace is now a necessity. We need to encourage food packaging that visibly carries health warning labels. In addition, Ministers of Finance will do well to (1) examine appropriate fiscal policy choices, such as "sin taxes" on tobacco and alcohol and understand the trade-offs involved; and (2) invest in social safety nets, especially health insurance coverage to prevent catastrophic health expenditure. In Nigeria, we are actively working on these.

Without action, we risk starting a vicious cycle where catastrophic health-care expenditure from rising noncommunicable diseases reverse economic and human development gains and plunge the middle class back into poverty. This scenario is not imagined. It is real and it is affecting many developing countries now. This trend needs to be tracked, halted, and, in fact, reversed. The issue is not to stop growth or the emergence of a middle class, both of which are economically and socially desirable, but to ensure that society is set on a trajectory of health and well-being required to sustain the newly attained prosperity.

Ngozi Okonjo-Iweala is the Minister of Finance and Coordinating Minister for the Economy of the Federal Republic of Nigeria and former Managing Director of the World Bank.

Chapter 71

Global Social Protection in Health

GORIK OOMS

It is time for humanity to accept its common responsibility for assuring the health of everyone, and to organize global social protection regimes accordingly.

Humans have always taken care of each other's health. Sharing food and water, nursing each other through illness—that was social protection for nomadic hunter-gatherer tribes. We can presume a dual motivation, a shared sense of communal belonging, and utility. A healthy tribe is better for all its members.

When tribes settled, when settlements became cities, when cities united to become nations, the circles of social protection expanded accordingly. In his *History of Public Health,* George Rosen mentions the sewage systems of sites excavated at Mohenjo-Daro and Harappa in India—built 4,000 years ago—as "activity connected with community health." Around the world, faith-based institutions have provided food and health care to the poor, supported by the rich, for centuries.

Circles of mutual social support have not always been geographically based. The medieval European guilds provided social protection by and for members. One of the oldest still-operational European private health insurers is the Benenden Healthcare Society. It was created in 1905 by post office employees to protect each other from the consequences of tuberculosis, an occupational hazard for postal workers. In his book *In Care of the State,* Abram de Swaan describes how present mutual health-care protection in Europe and the United States is rooted in initiatives that were originally local and linked to specific industries. He also describes how, in the long run, "even large and affluent corporations risked being burdened with more extensive disability and pension obligations than they had bargained for, burdens which threatened to weaken their competitive position in relation to companies that had established such schemes at a later day or not at all," and that, ultimately, only the state "could overcome the dilemmas of voluntary collective action by its coercive powers to levy taxes and impose membership."

What hope is there for global social protection in health—in the absence of a global government that could overcome the challenges of voluntary international collective action? The answer may depend on the global social protection regime one envisages. If one thinks of a single uniform regime, providing the same benefits for all, and collecting compulsory contributions in accordance with a single formula, the outlook is probably negative. However, if one thinks of a conglomerate of national and local schemes, each preserving their identity and governance, with only minimum standards and modest cross-subsidies, then 100 to 200 governments of sovereign states should be able to organize a system that serves their collective interests and responds to their citizens' increasing sentiment that we belong to "one world."

The Global Fund to Fight AIDS, Tuberculosis, and Malaria is a functioning example of a nascent global social protection in health regime. It is the result of a sense of belonging to a single humanity, captured by the slogan "We all have AIDS, if one of us does," and of the proven effectiveness of combating an infectious disease collectively, not country by country. Like Bob Deacon, Professor of Social Policy at the University of Sheffield, who wrote a seminal book on "Global Social Policy and Governance," I think that "steps towards a formal system of global redistribution that might eventually involve a Global Tax Authority and a Global Social Affairs Ministry will build upon firstly existing ad hoc mechanisms and secondly proposals for such mechanisms that are already within the global debate." The Global Fund is one such ad hoc mechanism on which we can build.

In the conclusion to *In Care of the State,* de Swaan draws parallels between the collectivization of social protection at the national level and the problem of global inequalities. He does not think the logical next wave of geographical expansion will come naturally, however, and he claims that there is currently no need for global collective action. On the contrary, I would argue that several historic decision-points are looming. Countries with more generous national social protection regimes will seek to protect themselves against trade competition from countries where they are nonexistent or less generous. This suggests the need for agreements on decent minimum levels, and cross-subsidies will be the logical and legitimate demand of countries expected to increase their present standards. To protect the world from the consequences of global warming, ecological efforts with economic consequences will be required from all countries, and countries with lower than average greenhouse gas emissions, lower than average economic development, and lower than average social protection can and will legitimately demand compensation.

It may take several decades before we can actually talk about a genuine global social protection regime. Meanwhile, those who see the moral imperative of addressing global health inequalities can already detect the contours of a nascent global social protection regime in existing mechanisms, and act accordingly.

Gorik Ooms is a human rights lawyer in the Department of Public Health at the Institute of Tropical Medicine Antwerp and former Executive Director of Médecins Sans Frontières Belgium.

Chapter 72

Inequities in Adolescent Health

ZULMA ORTIZ

Persisting challenges in adolescent health should be addressed by actively engaging teens in advocacy efforts and deliberative dialogues that will shape future programs and policies concerning their rights.

When is the best time in one's lifetime to reduce inequities in health?

Each stage of the life cycle offers opportunities to reverse poor health indicators; interventions at each stage will be different and will result in distinct outcomes. Then the question arises: what is the earliest stage at which a person can contribute not only to his or her own development processes, but also to reducing national and global inequities in health?

Adolescence is a stage of interaction, autonomy, and identity construction. This represents the perfect opportunity to engage adolescents in a variety of policy areas and processes to jointly build a development agenda to ensure the protection, respect, and fulfillment of their rights. It is known that teenagers face unique obstacles, including those directly concerned with discrimination on grounds of gender, culture, ethnicity, race, HIV/AIDS, and poverty—all preventing them from freely exercising their right to health. Gender stereotypes, social norms, and sexist attitudes make adolescents more vulnerable to sexual violence, teenage pregnancy, and HIV. Discrimination against LGBTI (lesbian, gay, bisexual, transgender, and intersex) teens can be a sign of alarm. Additionally, individuals in this age group often face restrictive laws that further impair their right to health. In many countries adolescents lack access to sexual and reproductive health services without parental consent. Other health problems affecting adolescents are poor nutrition among the poor and excluded groups, obesity, mental health problems, suicide, and non-intentional injuries such as deaths from violence or road traffic injuries. Lastly, it should be of highest concern that unlike child health, which is measured by universal indicators such as infant mortality, adolescent health currently has no standard measures of health.

Teens need to be informed and advocate for their health, but most importantly, they need to reinforce good values acquired at early ages and put into practice principles like solidarity and reciprocity. To support this change, we must produce evidence and mechanisms to mobilize and engage teenagers in a way that will allow them to feel part of the solution. This can be achieved through deliberative dialogues involving stakeholders representing government, academia, civil society, private sector, and, of course, adolescents themselves. These dialogues should generate structured policies, plans, and programs at various levels that work to reduce inequality and inequity in prioritized adolescent health indicators.

These deliberations would ultimately result in an agenda for public debate on significant equity gaps in adolescent health, with special emphasis on gender inequalities and the actions required to reduce inequities, with a description of roles and responsibilities to promote accountability and citizenship building.

People, especially teenagers, must understand that their participation in deliberative dialogue is necessary to set an agenda to achieve true global health. Outlining health priorities with an explicit, transparent, inclusive, and participatory approach is more likely to be accepted and implemented than when those decisions are in the hands of a few.

Zulma Ortiz is a health specialist with UNICEF Argentina and a Professor with Argentina's National Academy of Medicine.

Chapter 73

Sharing Financial Responsibilities

TRYGVE OTTERSEN

> We need to go beyond just setting goals and defining rights and ultimately move toward sharing responsibilities for health financing.

Goals for health and health services are important, but insufficient. Today there is near consensus on many general goals. The world has decided to reduce child mortality, strengthen national health systems, and be prepared for global pandemics. But agreements on goals like these have not been matched by agreements dictating who should finance the changes needed to achieve them. As a result, even universally agreed-upon goals are left unrealized.

We need a leap toward truly *shared* responsibilities for health financing. This means that every state, every individual, and every other actor contributes their fair share to the central goals of global health. They should do so out of self-interest, as risks and vulnerabilities are increasingly shared across populations. And they should do so for reasons of solidarity, justice, and human rights. This should be particularly clear for us living in countries where the financing of health services is already extensively shared. In our countries, it is widely held that risk should be pooled and that inability to pay should not be a barrier to health care. But then we must ask ourselves: how could this shared responsibility suddenly cease at national borders? To me, it seems impossible to justify today's abrupt shift: we take responsibility for financing even highly expensive, barely effective services for our fellow nationals, but take only limited responsibility for financing even cheap, lifesaving drugs for people abroad. National borders simply cannot carry this weight, and this is underscored by the fact that place of birth is as unchosen and arbitrary as race, color, and sex.

To see this even more clearly, you may imagine yourself in a situation where you do not know what country you live in. Then ask yourself how you want responsibilities for meeting health needs to be distributed across the world. I am quite sure you will not go for today's pattern. I believe you will want truly shared responsibilities, where everyone takes some responsibility for everyone else's health—to the degree that one can.

My generation of 20- and 30-year-olds is programmed to have this mindset of change. We travel—physically and virtually—more than any generation before us. Everyday we interact with people thousands of miles away. We care about the health of our Facebook friends, Skype contacts, and Twitter followers. The circle of concern is thus expanding, and the significance of national borders likely to pale.

But this will not happen on its own. All of us must actively attend to the idea of shared responsibilities and ensure that it pervades thinking and action in global affairs. We must explore the options for burden-sharing as thoroughly as we examine goals and rights. Policy formulation must more frequently involve clear assignment of responsibilities—even though that can be the hardest part. On this issue, the global health community has much to learn from the insights, successes, and failures in the field of environmental governance. By debating, cultivating, and refining the idea of shared responsibilities, we may eventually have a common language for the duty side of human rights and the responsibility side of global health goals.

Ultimately, we must seek a better overall framework for global health financing. It will need to specify how responsibilities are to be shared within and across three areas. The first is domestic financing of national health systems, where governments and other domestic actors collaborate in funding the health system within their own country. The second is external financing of national health systems, where wealthier actors outside poorer countries provide support. The third is joint financing of global public goods, where actors worldwide contribute to goods that will benefit everyone once they are provided.

Work on such frameworks has recently gained momentum, and many of the changes needed have already been identified. We must develop and seek agreement on clear targets for financing, as we already do for health outcome and health service goals. We must go beyond devising targets and ensure that actors are held accountable for meeting them. And we must focus intensely on the financing of global public goods, as such goods are becoming increasingly vital to global health. Among these goods are health information and surveillance systems, as well as research and development for new drugs and technologies. It is also clearer than ever that adequate health financing cannot be secured within the health sector alone. Action to overcome many key barriers, such as illicit financial flows and tax havens, is needed from other sectors. To secure sufficient funds, the global health community has to broaden its outlook and collaborate beyond its traditional frontiers.

If we are to succeed in creating a healthy future, we must continuously remind ourselves that goals and rights are only the first steps. Responsibilities must, and can be, better shared by us all.

Trygve Ottersen is a Postdoctoral Fellow at the University of Bergen and the Norwegian Institute of Public Health and was a member of the World Health Organization's Consultative Group on Equity and Universal Health Coverage.

Chapter 74

We're All in This Together

SEAN PENN

If we really want a healthy future, the barrier-free focus of emergency humanitarian responses must be carried through to prevention and long-term development.

Strapped into the pickup, hands gripping the stretcher as we rattle through Port-au-Prince searching desperately for the medication needed to treat diphtheria . . .

Rotten teeth extracted dark-ages-style from a patient whose head is resting on a beach ball . . .

Taking a switchblade to a canvas cot to allow diarrhea to flow from our latest patient directly into the open channel that lines our cholera treatment tent . . .

Over the past five years in Haiti, these and many similar scenarios have become commonplace. The great frustration is, of course, that each of these acute cases is preventable. With vaccines, toothbrushes, soap, and safe water, these tragedies-in-progress vanish. It seems so simple and straightforward. So you could be excused for thinking that what matters most for a healthy future is somehow different in countries like Haiti than for countries like the United States. The truth is, however, we're all in this together.

It wasn't the haunting images of piled bodies and pulverized neighborhoods that brought me to Haiti after the 2010 earthquake. I heard reports of parents helplessly holding the hands of their children during amputation procedures without so much as an Advil to dull their kids' pain. My son had just recovered from a near-fatal accident. I remembered how I had come to love that morphine drip that gave my son the relief that my handholding and his mother's couldn't. Hundreds of thousands dead and millions left homeless struck a chord, but the story that resonated with my own personal experience got me on that plane.

In the beginning, the mission was simple: save lives.

In moments like the earthquake—when the task is singular, all are dedicated, and there is no time for the pettiness that so often drags us down—we can get the best of humanity. Putting aside all their differences, the Government of Venezuela and the US military worked together to support my team of 30 international volunteers to deliver more than a quarter-of-a-million vials of pain medication to those most in need.

Over the past five years, the people of Haiti have taken incredible strides forward and the country has moved past the earthquake. Looking ahead, we must confront the fact that many natural disasters, like the acute medical cases mentioned earlier, can be prevented. It wasn't an earthquake that killed hundreds of thousands of people in January of 2010; it was decades of poverty and failed governance that allowed rubble-in-waiting to be hobbled together into the façade of a city, waiting to kill.

In response, our team grew and our mission evolved. Today, more than 300 full-time development professionals at J/P Haitian Relief Organization (HRO) are dedicated to saving lives and building sustainable programs with the Haitian people quickly and effectively. We are supporting families to create the resilient, sustainable, and prosperous communities necessary to prevent future shocks from spiraling into national crises. Our integrated, geographically focused programs bring medical care, education, livelihoods, protection, engineering, construction, and community programming together in one high-density, marginalized neighborhood in the center of Port-au-Prince.

Our medical program is working to address issues like access, cost, and information gaps. What we see is that where health teams like ours are active and work in partnership with the Haitian Ministry of Health, many people take advantage of the little things that go a long way:

vaccinations, deworming, vitamin A, dental hygiene, breastfeeding, handwashing, safe water, and chronic disease management. J/P HRO's labor and delivery team has safely brought more than 1600 babies into this world with an astounding 0% maternal mortality rate, and we continue to see about 2,000 patients every month. We are looking long-term, supporting communities as they lay their foundation for a healthy future.

The world demands more equitable care and more effective prevention for all. In emergencies, solutions can be clear and quick. We've learned that when artificial human barriers come down, priorities become clearer, action becomes more accurate, and our future goals quickly become our past accomplishments.

Today we must strive to bring that same level of dedication to prevention and long-term development. For a truly healthy future—for strong health systems, built infrastructure, and economic security that each person on our planet deserves—we're going to need to bring our best to bear. We must mobilize funding, ingenuity, dedication, will, and honesty to meet the world's demands. We can either condemn ourselves to perpetual cycles of emergency or we can look past the barriers that divide us and live the truth that we're all in this together.

Sean Penn is a two-time Academy Award-winning actor, founder of the J/P Haitian Relief Organization, and serves as Ambassador-at-Large of the Republic of Haiti.

Chapter 75

No Health without Rights

NAVANETHEM PILLAY

Health will only come into its own when human rights principles are integrated into health policy and programming at all levels.

In the language of the Basotho people of Southern Africa, the word for health, "bophelo," also means "life." It goes without saying that the dignity with which we live our lives is intimately bound to the health we either lack or enjoy. Poor health not only affects dignity and quality of life, but it also has a negative impact on the enjoyment of other human rights, such as the rights to education and work, which in turn will affect the right to an adequate standard of living. The attention paid globally to improving health outcomes testifies to the pivotal importance of health, a current example being the almost-universal support for including a health goal in the post-2015 development agenda.

Despite concerted efforts at both the international and domestic levels in this area, there is, regrettably, no shortage of health challenges to be overcome. To take maternal mortality as one example, the World Health Organization estimates that approximately 800 women die from preventable causes related to pregnancy and childbirth every day, that 99% of all maternal deaths occur in developing countries, and that maternal mortality is higher among women living in rural areas and in poorer communities. The tragedy is that most of these deaths are avoidable and poverty is arguably the factor most implicated in these outcomes. Thus, the poorer one is, the less likely one is to survive pregnancy and childbirth in good health or to deliver a healthy child. We also know that the majority of people living with HIV in low-income countries do not have access to treatment even as HIV is now widely considered to be a chronic condition or illness in the developed world due to the availability of antiretroviral medicines.

Clearly, discrimination is at the root of disparities in access to health care, both in terms of availability and quality of services. My strong conviction is that the one change most needed to improve health is the systematic implementation of a human rights–based approach to health at the country level.

By outcomes, I refer to the treatment and management of health problems, universal access to health care, and improvement in the underlying determinants of health.

When we discuss health in human rights terms, the international standard is that good quality health care, facilities, and goods should be available, accessible, and acceptable to all without discrimination. Furthermore, the beneficiaries of health services should be able to participate in the design and implementation of policies that affect them, and states should be accountable for meeting their obligation to respect, protect, and fulfill the right to heath. The human rights–based approach to health recognizes that the right to health does not only confer an entitlement to access to health care, it also requires that states pay attention to the underlying determinants of health, which include access to safe and potable water and adequate sanitation, an adequate supply of safe food and nutrition, and healthy occupational and environmental conditions. This calls for a commitment from governments that goes beyond ratifying treaties, and addresses the practical operationalization of their human rights obligations.

In addition to the sustainable improvement of health outcomes overall, applying human rights principles to the delivery of health care ensures that the vulnerable and marginalized are not excluded, and that other factors that impact the capacity to enjoy good health are addressed in a holistic manner. To complete this picture, this approach should be extended to the budgeting process, with states using all the resources available to them to ensure the progressive realization of all economic, social, and cultural rights, including health. Among other things, the efficient allocation and effective use of resources will provide an important safeguard against the worst effects of austerity measures in times of economic hardship.

Simply put, designing health programs without consideration for human rights is equivalent to responding to the plight of people living with HIV without providing access to adequate nutrition, which is crucial if treatment is to be successful. Such programs do not consider, in any depth, the responsibility of governments to be accountable to stakeholders and they do not address barriers to access to health care or the underlying determinants of health.

It is only when health policies, programs, and all aspects of health care are firmly founded on a human rights–based approach, with people squarely at the center, that the promise of healthy societies will be fully realized.

Navanethem Pillay is a former United Nations High Commissioner for Human Rights, Judge of the International Criminal Court, and President of the International Criminal Tribunal for Rwanda.

Chapter 76

No Magic Bullet

PETER PIOT

Beware of panaceas: we must face up to the complexity of global health challenges and encourage a multiplicity of approaches.

The search for any single solution to global health challenges is a chimera.

International cooperation is vital, but we must beware of the medico-technological hubris that we have a stock of magic-bullet solutions. The reality is we don't, even if the number and range of effective interventions in global health has grown significantly over recent decades.

The history of progress in health shows that, despite major advancements, our age-old struggle against infectious diseases is far from over. Malaria and tuberculosis are still rampant, HIV/AIDS continues to be a massive endemic burden, globalization of travel and food production has increased the threat of pandemics, and rising antimicrobial resistance risks reversing much of the progress made over the past 70 years.

The rise of chronic diseases presents even greater challenges, and sustainable solutions are far more likely to be found in prevention rather than cure. Our twenty-first-century lifestyle is not conducive to health, and policymakers must be bolder in promoting sustainable health and well-being. This means, where necessary, making structural interventions and taking a more proactive approach to discouraging unhealthy intakes (food, tobacco, and alcohol), while also developing transportation and a built environment that promote health, not disease. The health community must unreservedly embrace multi-sectoral action and consider involving a wider spectrum of scientific disciplines than has been employed to date, while pursuing technological innovation and inspiring confidence in lifesaving tools such as vaccines.

It will be crucial to sustain and expand what momentum we have in global health. Despite the scale and multiplicity of the challenges, let us not forget that the world has never seen so much progress in health as in the last few decades. Life expectancy has increased in nearly all countries, child mortality has decreased, as have HIV infection and mortality rates, and despite very recent setbacks, polio is close to elimination. The keys to these achievements have been economic development, local and global leadership, and international solidarity. Conversely, major inequalities in health persist within and between countries, and there have been reverses, especially in fragile states and conflict areas.

One lesson from the AIDS epidemic, and from development in general, is that the traditional "top-down" model does not work. This models involves researchers and funders from the global North expecting decision-makers in the South to implement "solutions" even when they are inappropriate to local context. Instead, we need a combination of top-down and bottom-up solutions, part of a larger understanding that the process is integral to the outcome.

Determinants of health are as much behavioral, social, and economic as they are biological or medical. Our challenge is to put health at the heart of government policy, and to couple it with adequate budgets and a commitment to change unhealthy cultures. We must be activists in health, but also in food, housing, environment, and research. In a world ruled by markets and political short-termism, such a broad citizens' movement will be essential to shift government and business priorities toward the long-term goal of sustainable health in a sustainable world.

Peter Piot is the Director of the London School of Hygiene and Tropical Medicine and former Executive Director of the Joint United Nations Programme on HIV/AIDS (UNAIDS).

Chapter 77

The Health Impact Fund

THOMAS POGGE

Creating a Health Impact Fund would greatly advance health around the world by promoting better use of available medicines, reducing health-care costs, and improving our arsenal of drugs.

We could achieve vastly better health worldwide by making better use of available medicines, while also redirecting pharmaceutical research and development (R&D) toward providing an arsenal of drugs more appropriate to the existing composition of the global disease burden.

The current system of pharmaceutical provision is shaped by Annex 1C of the World Trade Organization's Agreement on Trade-Related Aspects of Intellectual Property Rights. Under this agreement, innovators are rewarded through national patents that give them 20-year monopolies on the manufacture and sale of their new medicines.

Given existing great economic inequalities, this system leads to exorbitant markups that make patented medicines unaffordable to a majority of humankind. It also steers pharmaceutical research away from diseases concentrated among the poor, focusing instead on the development of maintenance drugs and close substitutes ("me-too drugs"). Additional inefficiencies arise from massive deadweight losses, wasteful expenditures on countless patents and patent litigation, competitive advertising, and counterfeits.

The system could be greatly improved by adding a second reward track for pharmaceutical innovators. The Health Impact Fund (HIF) is a proposed pay-for-performance scheme that would offer innovators the option to register any new medicine, thereby undertaking to make it available during its first 10 years on the market at or below cost. The registrant would further commit to allowing, at no charge, generic production and distribution of the product after expiry of this reward period.

In exchange, the registrant would participate during that decade in fixed annual reward pools divided among all registered products according to the individual drug's measured health impact. The size of these pools could be chosen to incentivize an appropriate number of important R&D projects. At $6 billion annually, the HIF might support some 25 new medicines at any time, with 2 or 3 entering and leaving each year.

Because the strength of the incentives depends on secure long-term funding, the reward pools would ideally be financed through a sizable endowment fed from contributions by states (proportional to their gross national income), international agencies, civil society organizations, foundations, corporations, individuals, and estates.

The HIF would foster the development of new high-impact medicines and, in particular, turn the now-neglected diseases of the poor into some of the most lucrative pharmaceutical R&D opportunities. It would avoid the bias that currently favors maintenance drugs by fully rewarding health gains achieved by preventative and curative drugs. It would also discourage the development of me-too drugs by rewarding them only insofar as they produce health gains beyond those achieved by their similar predecessors.

The HIF would promote access to registered medicines by limiting their price to the lowest feasible cost of manufacture and distribution. Registrants would often benefit from selling to the very poor at extremely low prices—even below cost—because they would receive increased health impact rewards.

The HIF would motivate registrants to care not about mere sales but about health gains. Registrants would focus their marketing on patients who can really benefit from their product, regardless of their socioeconomic status. Registrants would have a stake in ensuring that their medicines are widely available, competently prescribed, and optimally used. Additional dramatic efficiency gains would arise from avoiding deadweight losses (no markups) and counterfeiting: with the genuine item widely available at or below cost, making and selling fakes is unprofitable. Finally, the HIF would also avert much costly litigation: generic firms would lack incentives to compete, and registrants would lack incentives to suppress generic products. Registrants might therefore not even bother to file for patents in many national jurisdictions.

The HIF requires an affordable, consistent, and reliable methodology for measuring the health impact of new medicines across diverse countries, patients, and diseases. Assessment of what a new drug adds to the length and quality of human lives would be based on data from clinical trials, on pragmatic trials in real-life settings, on tracking randomly selected medicines to their end users, and on statistical analysis of sales data as correlated with data about the global disease burden. These estimates would necessarily be rough, at least in the early years. But so long as any errors are random, or at least not exploitable by registrants, HIF incentives would be only minimally disturbed.

By providing access to important pharmaceutical innovations at rock-bottom prices, the HIF would easily pay for itself. Through lower drug prices, taxpayers would realize offsetting savings in national health systems, insurance premiums, direct pharmacy purchases, and foreign aid. We all would benefit from reductions in counterfeiting, wasteful litigation, and excessive marketing. By stimulating development of important but currently unprofitable medicines, by making new high-impact medicines much more widely accessible, and by encouraging efforts to ensure that medicines are optimally used, the HIF would greatly reduce the global disease burden and thereby produce large medical cost savings and productivity gains. Contributions to the HIF would produce vastly greater health gains per dollar than the $600 billion humankind is now spending each year on patented medicines.

Thomas Pogge is the founding Director of the Global Justice Program and Leitner Professor of Philosophy and International Affairs at Yale University, and is a Professor of Philosophy at King's College London, University of Oslo, and University of Central Lancashire.

Chapter 78

Value-Based Health-Care Delivery

MICHAEL E. PORTER

Measuring and reporting standardized outcomes per condition across the globe would lead to unprecedented health-care transformation.

The problems in health care are well known, and there is vast literature documenting the problems, abuses, and faulty incentives in the system. Improving insurance coverage, elevating the role of consumers in decision-making, identifying and implementing evidence-based practice guidelines, and harnessing the promise of information technology—these are all ideas that have been explored and implemented to some extent. However, work that examines the essential purpose and nature of competition in health-care delivery, and which addresses the strategy, organization, and measurement for health-care delivery organizations, has been lacking.

I believe that the transformation of health care must start by understanding that the fundamental goal of any health-care organization must be to improve value for patients, defined as the health outcomes achieved per dollar spent. Improving value for patients is the only goal that can unite the interests of all health system participants, and it is the only real solution to the challenges we currently face in providing health care. Value improvement will require major changes in the way health care is delivered, measured, and reimbursed, not just incremental improvement.

Today, more and more health systems around the world are focusing on the concept of value. In nearly every advanced economy, restructuring competition, transparency, and payment around value is recognized as the only way to actually slow the growth of medical costs. Yet progress is still frustratingly slow. This is because, in most areas of medicine, there is no consensus on what defines value, which starts with the outcomes that matter most to patients. This lack of a comprehensive framework for measuring and reporting outcomes is the single biggest impediment to rapid restructuring in health systems. Without transparency on outcomes, progress is slow in improving quality, and we lack the most essential tool needed to drive appropriate cost reduction. Without outcomes, the move to value-based reimbursement approaches is retarded. And competition remains a zero-sum fight for resources and market power.

I believe that measuring and reporting standardized outcomes by condition across the globe would help catalyze a global movement toward value-based health care and lead to unprecedented health-care transformation. Any provider could benchmark their performance and compete to deliver outcomes on par with the best in the world. Any patient could make a more informed decision on where to seek care, even across borders. Furthermore, new payment models based on outcomes could be developed and replicated around the world.

The transformation to value-based health-care delivery will take time, but the process is now underway. I invite you to participate in this movement, access the growing knowledge on value-based approaches in many medical fields, and join the community of practitioners who are pursuing the fundamental purpose that attracted most of us to health care in the first place.

Michael E. Porter is the Bishop William Lawrence University Professor and Director of the Institute for Strategy and Competitiveness at Harvard Business School.

Chapter 79

Acknowledging Ignorance

ESTHER DUFLO

We must acknowledge that we know very little about what might work in global health and set out to rigorously test ideas before they are scaled up.

The biggest obstacle to improving global health is that so many of us are convinced that we know what is the biggest obstacle to improving it. And, to boot, that we have the solution for it.

These great ideas are generally perfectly sensible and generous: free health care; beneficiary oversight; free medications; catastrophic health insurance; the right to health; improved stoves; handwashing campaigns; arsenic awareness campaigns; toilets for everyone . . .

The problem is that most of these ideas are untested. And, when they are tested, they do not always deliver what is initially expected. Take improved stoves, for example. Tens of thousands of them were circulated in India in the 1980s. Villagers had no interest in them and they soon broke down. The remnants of many of them can still be seen in the fields. In the 2000s, the idea, as ideas do, reemerged. The stoves, we were told, were now so much better, and there would surely be a high demand for them. Without testing this proposition, international donors set themselves the challenge to "foster the adoption of clean cookstoves and fuels in 100 million households by 2020." I too was entirely convinced that better cookstoves would have large health effects and, with some collaborators, I set out to demonstrate that they would also have an effect on productivity in Orissa, India. But, as many others have also shown since then, while the design of the stoves had improved, the demand for them still appears to be very low. We continued to face the issue that, in realistic field conditions, the stoves were neither used much nor maintained. The project concluded with the lesson that since the stoves were not in use, there was no impact on health.

I had a similarly sad experience with catastrophic health insurance. A microfinance partner we worked with attempted to bundle microcredit and health insurance. Our idea was to test whether knowing that they now have insurance against the worst health crises would encourage households to take more risk. What we found is that many households faced with the choice to get insurance or to give up on microcredit just gave up microcredit! This is how much they valued insurance.

In both cases, there were reasons for the failures, of course. But they were not obvious before we did the research. In both instances we tested ideas that were widely believed to make perfect sense and implemented them earnestly given the constraints in the field.

The general lesson is that we have so little understanding about health behavior and beliefs that we have no idea how a particular innovation may be received until we try it in the field and give ourselves the chance to estimate its impact. Free malaria medication will spur resistance if people take malaria medication even if they test negative for malaria (they do). Anti-arsenic campaigns will kill babies if people switch from arsenic-contaminated (but clean) wells to dirty shallow pools (they do). And so on.

Fortunately we know what to do: after all, we are used to measuring the impact of new medications with rigorous randomized control trials. The same can be done with processes, tools, and policies. Any new idea presents the potential to learn a little more and, in a few years, we may indeed have 100 *really* good ideas to improve global health.

Esther Duflo is a Founder and Director of the Abdul Latif Jameel Poverty Action Lab and the Abdul Latif Jameel Professor of Poverty Alleviation and Development Economics at the Massachusetts Institute of Technology.

Chapter 80

Universal Ideas/Local Institutions

MARIANA MOTA PRADO

We must learn how to best design institutions adapted to local contexts so they can effectively spread universally helpful ideas.

What has caused the dramatic improvements in global health witnessed over the past century? Some may say money, as wealth is often correlated with better health. Indeed, richer countries generally have better health indicators. However, this is not always the case. The United Nations' Human Development Index (HDI) has often shown that there is no perfect correlation between income and other development indicators, such as health and education. For example, Chile, Cuba, and Vietnam fare better on health and education (and in the overall HDI ranking) than economically comparable countries, whereas Angola, Bahrain, and the United States do worse. The trend toward a "grand convergence in global health" that some scholars have identified has not thus far been accompanied by a convergence in global wealth. Thus, improvement in health is not necessarily a result of economic growth or increased wealth per capita.

If wealth does not account fully for these improvements, what else could explain the significant progress achieved in global health over the last few decades? Ideas have played an important role in this process. An enhanced body of scientific knowledge has promoted changes in daily habits (e.g., handwashing), the creation of devices to prevent disease transmission (e.g., malaria bed nets and condoms), and inventions that have vastly improved health care (e.g., vaccines). These ideas and the inventions associated with them have been disseminated around the world, helping to improve health outcomes even in countries that have not witnessed significant increases in wealth. One of the most dramatic examples is Haiti. Between 1950 to 2002, this country has experienced a decline in income from $1,000 to $700 per capita, while its infant mortality has dropped from 20% to less than 8%.

Spreading these ideas as quickly and effectively as possible requires functional institutions at the national level. For instance, handwashing requires easy access to clean water. Other recommendations for personal hygiene that can vastly improve health indicators depend on the existence of a functional sanitation system. In some cases, developing countries' lack of systems to provide clean water and/or sanitation services is because of a lack of resources. However, in many (if not most) cases, the biggest problem is the lack of effective institutions to employ existing resources effectively. Indeed, in many cases, an increase in resources such as through extractive industries or foreign aid does not translate into improvements in service provision because of inefficient or corrupt national institutions.

Reforming dysfunctional institutions at the national level is the biggest challenge facing global health today. Attempts to create effective institutions in developing countries have been met with significant obstacles, such as political resistance, cultural differences, and path dependence. Most importantly, effective institutional design is highly context dependent and, as the evidence shows, reforms are unlikely to be successful if based on universal blueprints. As a consequence, efforts to spread universally helpful ideas will only be successful if they are based on highly context-specific strategies. Only local institutional knowledge will allow these universal ideas to reach the four corners of the world.

Mariana Mota Prado is Associate Dean and Associate Professor at the University of Toronto's Faculty of Law.

Chapter 81

From Pulse to Planet

K. SRINATH REDDY

Human health is integrally related to planetary health; recognition of this interdependence can advance health within a framework that respects both sustainable development and intergenerational equity.

The health of humans is integrally and inextricably linked to the health of the whole planet. Humankind can be assured of good health and well-being only if it values the harmonious interdependence of all life forms and ecosystems that compose the planet, across the porous boundaries of time and territory. Embedding human health in the construct of planetary health will not only promote human well-being in its biological and social dimensions, but will also protect our environment and move our civilization to a higher moral plane of commitment to intergenerational equity.

To any thoughtful student or practitioner of public health, it is now abundantly clear that a reductionist approach is extremely limited in explaining the factors that protect health or the processes that cause disease. If nothing else, the revelation that trillions of friendly bacteria in our gut and elsewhere in the body constitute a microbiome that protects us in many ways should evoke humility and awe at the interdependence of life forms.

The planet provides for interactions of humans with its vast biodiversity and varied components of its physical environment, which in turn shape the state of human health. Well beyond the speculative associations suspected over past millennia, robust science now provides convincing proof of the close links between our physical environment and health. We now understand how climate change can affect health through heat effects, extreme weather events, vectors that transmit infectious disease, migration of climate refugees, and impact on agriculture and nutrition. We now live in a world where our agriculture and food systems are degrading the environment and an endangered environment is threatening food security.

Meanwhile, industrial-scale livestock production generates half of the world's methane emissions while setting up a conveyor belt for potential animal-to-human transmission of zoonotic pathogens. Apart from being highly water intensive, such factory farming of livestock divests land from traditional crops for disproportionate growing of grains and then diverts those grains for animal feed. This process exacerbates food and nutrition insecurity for many people. Excess meat and corn production also raise the risk of chronic diseases and agricultural practices that are insensitive to national or global nutrition needs. Ultimately, this results in an overabundance of a few commercially favored crops that do not provide the dietary diversity needed for healthy nutrition. Deforestation resulting from distorted agricultural priorities and damaging practices undermines the environment, with further adverse effects on health and nutrition.

Even the environmental effects of tobacco should challenge our conscience, besides its horrendous health effects. Apart from killing 100 million humans in the last century and threatening to kill a billion more over the next 100 years, it contributes to deforestation through the burning of wood for "curing" the leaf and extensive use of paper for packaging. A modern cigarette machine uses four miles of paper per hour. In other words, a tree is killed for every 300 cigarettes smoked. High levels of pesticide and water needed by tobacco plants also pose threats to planetary resources. It is also unconscionable that nearly four million hectares of arable land are wasted on a killer crop while large parts of the world are haunted by hunger.

The recognition of interconnectivity and interdependence among all life and ecosystems should bring greater commitment to global health as a shared value. Initiatives such as universal health coverage, worldwide access to essential drugs, "one health" eco-surveillance, regulation of unhealthy foods and beverages, virus sharing for vaccine production, and improving global governance for health cannot succeed without a spirit of solidarity and a sense of common survival. The concept of human health as an integral part of planetary health can liberate us from the narrow and erroneous definition of health as an individual attribute that devolves upon individual responsibility.

We owe it to future generations to not deprive them of their right to live in a healthy society supported by a healthy planet. This moral imperative must motivate us to create a legacy of a tobacco-free, environment-friendly, health-promoting society where global nutrition needs guide agriculture and food systems, and access to health and health care are assured for all in a value framework that enshrines equity and prizes quality. Is that a utopian dream? I do not think so. I believe this is the only way human civilization can survive and prosper, to enjoy good health and well-being among the many gifts that acting on this transformative insight can bring.

K. Srinath Reddy is the President of the Public Health Foundation of India, former President of the World Heart Federation, and former Head of the Department of Cardiology at All India Institute of Medical Sciences.

Chapter 82

A War on Tuberculosis

ZAIN RIZVI

Given that global health crises are deadlier than armed conflicts, we should attend to them, at minimum, with the same zeal that defines our response to other unacceptable realities.

With escalating conflict in Syria, Afghanistan, and Iraq, 2012 was an especially violent year. As soldiers took to the streets, brutal scenes of armed rebellions and government crackdowns stunned people all over the world. In response, many in the West took to the streets too, as protestors and activists. The United Nations raised concerns about the growing civilian death toll.

One of the most deadly clashes of the year, however, received little attention.

Tuberculosis killed more people than all the wars that year combined, 13 times over. A disease of the lungs, tuberculosis has robbed human potential and attacked human dignity like few other killers in history. Yet there were no mass protests, no strongly worded United Nations resolutions, no pundits expressing outrage for this battle against bacteria.

Why do we give such little attention to these conflicts? We only have to look at the hysteria surrounding the recent Ebola outbreak to see that our response to global health crises is limited to the extent that we feel afraid or threatened.

One reason is that we tend to focus on the new and urgent. A deadly incursion by an insurgent group grabs our attention because it disturbs the status quo in a concentrated burst of violence. In contrast, tuberculosis epidemics progress slowly, ravaging communities over months. Tragedy prolonged no longer seems as tragic. More fundamentally, tuberculosis epidemics half a world away do not hold our attention because they do not disturb the norm—in a perverted sense, they *are* the status quo.

These twisted expectations expose the root of our apathy: we perceive military conflicts as preventable man-made evils, but global health crises as inevitable, as natural, as parts of the world beyond our control. Through this narrative, we excuse and normalize the preventable suffering and deaths of millions of innocent people. How else could we accept living with the fact that tuberculosis alone could orphan up to 50 million children—civilians by any measure—in the next five years?

In the story that we tell ourselves, we first lessen our burden by deferring to the natural order of things. Tuberculosis may be horrible but death is inevitable; nature is simply taking its course. Yet there is nothing natural or inevitable about the actions people take that allow the bacteria to thrive. *Mycobacterium tuberculosis* rarely acts alone. Instead, it is supported by poorly trained physicians and nurses who misdiagnose and mistreat the disease; community leaders who perpetuate stigma and a culture of fear; pharmaceutical company executives who decide to pursue research and development for drugs targeting erectile dysfunction over tuberculosis; and ultimately politicians who prioritize sexy short-term projects over investment and development in health systems.

Second, we tell ourselves that the situation lies beyond our control. We couldn't even make a difference if we tried. But this part of the narrative is also largely false: global health crises are often both preventable and man-made. Cost-effective solutions exist for many global health challenges. And while the tuberculosis infection may not be man-made, the lack of appropriate response and care, which fuel the global health crisis, is completely under our control. If held accountable, a range of actors—governments, civil society, and industry groups—could catalyze significant improvements in well-being globally. Certainly our ability to press for pro-health policies has a greater chance of making a difference than advocating for military intervention, or the lack thereof, to mediate centuries-old ethnic and sectarian divisions.

The stories we tell ourselves to help us feel better are not only patently false, but also deeply unjust. Death may be inevitable but suffering is not, nor is depriving someone the chance to live a rich and fulfilling life. The shrieks of a child who has lost her mother do not vary according to whether bullets or bacteria killed her, no matter how "natural" the mother's death may seem.

A War on Tuberculosis is no less needed than a War on Terror. What is required from us, then, is to recognize that global health is a cause worth fighting for, and to attend to these crises with the same empathy and zeal that define our response to other fundamentally unacceptable realities of our time. Our attention is the least we can give.

Zain Rizvi is a JD Candidate at Yale Law School and a Student Fellow with the Global Health Justice Partnership at Yale University.

Chapter 83

Universal Health Coverage

JUDITH RODIN

Universal health coverage offers us the greatest hope for improving health worldwide.

Six years ago, during a visit to a slum in Bangladesh, I watched as a young pregnant woman had her hypertension diagnosed through a mobile application and then received lifesaving medication. It took under three minutes. The procedure was provided by the BRAC Manoshi program free of charge, but would have otherwise been prohibitively expensive. She would have had to make the choice between treatment or financial burden, and she probably wouldn't have gotten a diagnosis at all.

This was the moment that I began to truly understand the potential of universal health coverage—providing every individual with the basic health services they need, without the risk of financial hardship. When the idea of universal health coverage was first introduced to the global community, the popular wisdom was that it couldn't be done. We would have neither the political will nor the resources to make such an ambitious goal a reality, particularly in developing and emerging economies.

But since 2008, more than 70 countries have approached the World Health Organization to request technical assistance in moving forward on universal health coverage. Countries are finding that access to quality, affordable health services not only improves people's lives and productivity, it also strengthens their economies. In fact, a recent Lancet Commission, chaired by Larry Summers, concluded that about 24%

of the economic growth in low- and middle-income countries between 2000 and 2011 was because of improved health.

Now, a movement has built among global and national actors, leading to the passage of a United Nations resolution in December 2012 to make universal health coverage a key global health objective. Today, dozens of countries are pursuing that goal, with many already showing success. In Rwanda, for example, in 1999, before the country adopted universal health coverage, only one percent of the population had health coverage. By 2012, that number had skyrocketed to 90%.

But the progress of individual countries is only one piece of empirical evidence that gives us hope that universal health coverage is the next big thing in global health. The other, perhaps more telling than the first, is that countries are coming together and learning from each other's progress.

Why is this important? Because it shows the appetite for universal health coverage is high, and the commitment to implementation matches this rigor. Countries are building health programs to fit the pressing needs of their people, rather than applying a one-size-fits-all solution, ensuring that universal health coverage is more than a passing trend.

We still have a good deal of work to do to ensure that health coverage is not just universal but equitable—that everyone, regardless of race or gender or income or geography, receives the quality health services they need at a price they can afford. But we have proven that big dreams matched with bold action can turn trends into transformations, and I believe that millions, like the woman I met in Bangladesh, will reap its rewards.

Judith Rodin is President of the Rockefeller Foundation and former President of the University of Pennsylvania and Provost of Yale University.

Chapter 84

Regulating Antimicrobials

JOHN-ARNE RØTTINGEN

We need global agreements to promote access to and effectiveness of antimicrobials as public and collective goods, which can be achieved through an international treaty.

My home country of Norway learned about the harms of overexploiting common-pool resources the hard way. In the 1960s we almost fully depleted our herring and cod stocks, and before that we contributed to overwhaling of the Southern Ocean. We eventually realized that strong regulations are needed to protect common-pool resources that are finite in supply and limit people's use of them. We solved many tragedies of the commons this way. For example, quotas were imposed to limit overfishing in Norwegian waters and international treaties were signed to prevent whales' extinction.

Today we face a new common-pool resource challenge in need of a strong regulatory response: the overexploitation of antimicrobials. This is vital because bacterial and viral infections remain one of the greatest threats to human health globally. While better housing, hygiene, and sanitation have contributed to reducing this threat, it was not until the advent of antimicrobials that we were able to treat and control infections. Unfortunately, the effectiveness of these drugs is not an everlasting good. Resistance to antimicrobials gradually and inevitably emerges, rendering them ineffective. The rate at which this happens is dependent on how we use them. Overuse and misuse will greatly shorten the time we have to treat life-threatening infections. Today more than 100,000 patients die worldwide each year due to antimicrobial resistance, and deaths are just the tip of the iceberg. Effective antimicrobials are also necessary to support modern medical procedures like implants and transplants, and resistance threatens to make these lifesaving treatments impossible in the near future. In other words, the effectiveness of antimicrobials is a limited common-pool resource that we need to manage much better.

The other side of our antimicrobial dilemma is that lack of access to these drugs still causes more deaths—at least 10 times more—than their misuse. Indeed, almost 100 years after the first discovery of antimicrobials, deaths from infections should have been history by now. Access to such essential medicines is rightfully considered a human right. And while several international initiatives currently promote access to antimicrobials—including the Global Fund to Fight AIDS, Tuberculosis, and Malaria, and UNITAID—these efforts surely need to be strengthened and expanded to ensure universal access to all lifesaving drugs.

Antimicrobials are not naturally renewable resources, though. As existing drugs develop resistance, we need to renew the stock of antimicrobials through time-consuming and costly research and innovation. In the pharmaceutical industry, such efforts and investments are rewarded through high prices in a patent-protected monopoly period. However, antimicrobials are a unique commodity, and there are two reasons high prices are a bad thing. First, we do not want lack of affordability to be a barrier for access. Second, we do not want profits from high prices and increased sales to be an incentive for encouraging overuse instead of preservation. Given that the pharmaceutical industry is driven by profits, stakeholders are increasingly calling for innovation models that delink the rewards for innovation from the number of antimicrobial units sold. Several such mechanisms that can incentivize development of new antimicrobials and nurture innovative competition have been proposed. Some are currently being tested. These models can turn antimicrobials into global public goods that are financed collectively across countries, much like individuals pay for national public goods through tax systems.

Antimicrobials are a global resource, and resistance to them can be seen as a global externality. Three important functions of the global health system are to produce global public goods, to manage externalities, and to provide solidarity. In the context of antimicrobials, we have seen piecemeal efforts to do all this through product development partnerships, the pandemic influenza preparedness system, and global health financing initiatives like Gavi, the Vaccine Alliance. However, to effectively preserve antimicrobials and slow the development of resistance, we need one concerted mechanism that encompasses these three interdependent functions. We need universal access to protect lives, but expansion of access must be achieved through responsible utilization. Better managed and more regulated markets are likewise prerequisites for large public investments into or incentives for research and development. Such investments are needed to develop new antimicrobials through novel, internationally collective innovation models. We need an innovative global agreement that can encompass all these issues and interests in one negotiation process, and then hold states accountable to their commitment. An International Treaty on Access to and Effectiveness of Antimicrobials would be the first of its kind to jointly regulate those three functions, and one of the changes most needed for sustained protection of population health.

John-Arne Røttingen is Director of Infectious Disease Control at the Norwegian Institute of Public Health, Professor of Health Policy at the University of Oslo, and Adjunct Professor of Global Health and Population at the Harvard T.H. Chan School of Public Health.

Chapter 85

Who Will Lead?

SIMON RUSHTON

Global health faces a looming crisis of leadership; where will the next generation of global health leaders come from, and will they be any more representative than the last?

Over the last two decades global health has enjoyed something of a golden age, occupying an unprecedented position on high-level international political agendas. This has not come about by accident, but as the result of political momentum generated and sustained by those who have exercised leadership.

These leaders have generally not been from medical or public health backgrounds or institutions. Back in 2006, an article in *Science* by Jon Cohen identified "the rocker Bono, matinee idols Angelina Jolie and Richard Gere, former US presidents Jimmy Carter and Bill Clinton, U.K. Prime Minister Tony Blair, U.N. Secretary-General Kofi Annan, and economist-cum-firebrand Jeffrey Sachs" as being particularly influential, with Bill and Melinda Gates "at the forefront." Whatever list we might individually compile, it is clear that global health leadership is about the exercise of power, and the ability to influence those with power. Medical and public health expertise plays an important role to be sure, but statesmen, celebrities, and super-rich philanthropists are the ones who can really "make things happen."

The leaders we have had reflect a particular time in the development of "global health" as a distinct field of international concern. They are from the generation that witnessed the emergence of HIV/AIDS in the West and the disease's catastrophic impact (and the impact of other humanitarian crises such as famine and conflict) across sub-Saharan Africa in the 1980s and 1990s. By the turn of the millennium, they found themselves in positions that enabled them to take action and devote significant resources to addressing global health challenges. They focused their efforts on infectious diseases, especially HIV/AIDS.

While there have been many failures and much to criticize along the way, what *has* undoubtedly been achieved is a high level of global political prioritization for health. As this generation of leaders moves on, however, and as the nature of the global disease burden changes, we should be worried about whether or not a new cohort of powerful global health advocates will emerge to take their place. This is particularly concerning given the radically different political and economic context we now inhabit compared to the boom years that preceded the financial crisis.

We should also be worried about the profile of our future leaders. Those of the last 20 years have been, for the most part, white, male, and from (or at least educated in) the global North. As such they reflect the global distribution of power and resources, but they are entirely unrepresentative of those who suffer the highest burden of disease in the world today. Our leaders are the beneficiaries of an unjust world, not those to whom health equity is denied. Though we have seen examples of real change brought about by grassroots activists and politicians in the developing world, they have rarely been given the chance to shape what happens at the global level. It is no wonder that some are beginning to ask whether global health is neocolonialist. We urgently need to find ways to make global politics (in health and all other fields) more democratic, and to make accountability real.

We are facing a potential leadership crisis of two dimensions. Will those with the ability to "make things happen" in the future exercise their power and influence in pursuit of global health objectives? If not, the "golden age" will truly be over.

If they do, how can we ensure that leadership in global health is exercised in ways that are reflective of the needs, wishes, and priorities of those in whose name "global health interventions" are made? This is a real challenge of leadership: to transform "global health" into a genuinely *global* endeavor that rests upon the solid foundations of a recognition of rights and the pursuit of justice, not the more shaky footings of individual altruism, political self-interest, and passing celebrity-endorsed fad.

Simon Rushton is a Faculty Research Fellow with the Department of Politics at the University of Sheffield.

Chapter 86

The Rwandan Consensus

RICHARD SEZIBERA

We can learn much about improving global health by looking at how Rwanda successfully reformed its health-care system.

Global health has come a very long way, between yesterday and today. And yet, the ideas that have led to so many remarkable successes in recent decades have been relatively simple. Having been Rwanda's Minister of Health during a time of revolutionary health-care reforms, I can vouch for this personally. After the genocide against the Tutsi in 1994, Rwandan life expectancy at birth was estimated to be 35 years. Today, it is 64.5 years and increasing. Maternal mortality was 1,500 per 100,000 live births in 2000; in 2014, it is estimated to be 340 per 100,000 live births, highlighting a 76% percent decline in maternal mortality and putting the country ahead of the Millennium Development Goal target for 2015.

Yet when I became Minister, I was told by experts that Rwanda—and the rest of Africa—would not be able to achieve global targets in the reduction of maternal mortality. They said that this goal would require near-impossible health interventions, but I was not convinced. Today, Rwanda is in competition with Switzerland in terms of equitable maternal care.

At the turn of the century, others claimed that antiretrovirals would not work in Africa because Africans were incapable of appreciating the concept of time and would not adhere to the strict antiretroviral schedules. Rwanda's success, replicated across the continent, is as strong a rejoinder as could be imagined. Today, 83% of patients on antiretrovirals have an undetectable viral load, an indicator that they do actually take the drugs on schedule. Over 91% of Rwandese who require antiretrovirals actually have them. The comparative figure for the United States is 75%.

So how did my war-torn country become the poster child for successful health-care reform? At the micro level, the solutions to existing health provision challenges were obvious. We needed to organize care around the patient, and the nexus between medicine and technology allowed us to do so. Device connectivity, geo-connectivity, and bio-connectivity, properly harnessed, can, for example, allow us to track maternal mortality in resource-constrained environments. In Rwanda, it allows the Minister to receive real-time updates on maternal deaths. Health-care providers and communities know they will have to carry out maternal death audits, encouraging them to invest in the simple interventions that reduce preventable deaths. But it also allows opportunities for moving the aged out of impersonal retirement homes, providing home- and community-based care, monitored through a network of intelligent bio-connectivity. At the global level, however, the "Rwanda Consensus" must drive the agenda. This involves six imperatives.

First, health must be accepted as an enforceable basic human right, with the requisite constitutional guarantees. Second, leadership will be critical. In Rwanda, the President is the Minister of Health par excellence, making sure the requisite resources are available—above the Abuja target of 15% of annual national budgets—and insisting on accountability for resources and results, with a relentless focus on equity. There is no substitute for this at the local and global levels. Third, we must take on these challenges with international solidarity. Perhaps no global partnership shows the importance of smart global investments in health better than Gavi, the Vaccine Alliance. By 2015, Gavi partners will have immunized half a billion children. That is impressive in its own right, but Gavi also provides a rate of return of 18% by 2020, similar to the returns for primary education. In the next decades, global partnerships will reduce long-term illness, long-term disability, and increase savings for health systems and families. Fourth, we must invest in innovation. In East Africa, under-5 mortality has decreased by 44%

and maternal mortality rates have been halved, thanks in part to innovations made possible by increased mobile telephone and fiber-optic penetration. Rwandan community health workers have access to information and ambulance services, and Kenyan mothers have access to finance through M Pesa. This is frontier territory and the nexus between medicine and technology will revolutionize the health landscape. Fifth, we need accountability measures for resources and results. In the East African Community, the Open Health Initiative promotes accountability around results and resource allocation. This effort has facilitated knowledge sharing and sometimes even friendly regional competition to incentivize political action. Through a score card and regional database, leaders have visibility on progress against key targets. Governments can compare program performance and spending to identify and learn from high-performing programs.

Lastly, we must prioritize universal access to health. The goal must be to ensure that all people everywhere obtain the health services they need without catastrophic household financial spending. This will have to be achieved through legislation, regulation, and taxation. We know that investments in health may account for as much as 24% of economic growth in low- and middle-income countries. Providing health to an extra two billion people will require renewed commitments to financial solidarity and a relentless focus on more health for every penny spent. The barrier to this lofty goal is neither lack of knowledge nor unavailability of resources. It is a lack of determined leadership. Today we really need leadership that is sufficiently determined to break through narrow parochial concerns.

It seems to me that the next few decades provide an unparalleled opportunity to invest in those interventions we know work. The challenge is enormous, and we shall have to feed and provide quality health care for an additional two billion people. It will require global solidarity, strict accountability measures, and strong leadership. But as we learned in Rwanda, it is possible.

Richard Sezibera is the Secretary-General of the East African Community and former Minister of Health of Rwanda.

Chapter 87

Ending Preventable Child Death

RAJIV SHAH

Preventing child mortality is a grand challenge, but it's within reach.

Since the dawn of humanity, child death has been a tragic fact of life. A century ago, just one country—Sweden—had an infant mortality rate below 10%. Today, fewer than 20 countries have an infant mortality rate *above* 10%. From 1990 to 2010, human ingenuity and entrepreneurship reduced child mortality rates by half—giving millions of children the opportunity to survive and thrive. Thanks to this remarkable progress, we stand within reach of a world that was once unimaginable: a world without preventable child death.

Yet, the challenge remains immense. Every year, more than 6 million children still die before their fifth birthday—many of them in developing countries. If we hope to end preventable child death within the next two decades, it will take more than new medicines. It will take a global effort—one grounded in coordinated action, targeted investments, and measurable results.

That is why, in 2012, the United States, Ethiopia, and India, along with UNICEF, hosted the *Child Survival: Call to Action* conference and launched *A Promise Renewed*, a global movement rallying the world behind a new approach to end preventable child death. It was a powerful moment, as 178 countries and more than 460 civil society and faith organizations stepped forward to join this mission.

Since then, nearly a dozen countries have launched their own local calls to action, set national targets, and created evidence-based report cards and action plans to focus resources in the most vulnerable regions. Within the US Agency for International Development, we have narrowed our focus to where the need is most acute: in the 24 countries that represent more than 70% of maternal and child deaths.

Two years later, we reconvened the global community at *Acting on the Call* to take stock of our progress. Empowered by this more innovative, unified, and data-driven approach, countries that had long struggled with high child mortality are beginning to deliver critical results.

For example, India targeted its efforts in the 184 districts with the highest rates of child death and has cut child mortality by more than 6% in two years. In the Democratic Republic of the Congo, we are integrating once separate systems for treating malaria, pneumonia, and other deadly illnesses into a single health program. In two years, the rate of child death dropped by 18% in targeted areas. Ethiopia—once one of the most dangerous places for a child to be born—created a cadre of 38,000 frontline health extension workers to reach vulnerable children and expectant women. In 2013, Ethiopia reached the Millennium Development Goal of reducing child mortality by two-thirds.

This kind of progress is only possible by harnessing a new model of development—one grounded in country leadership, innovative financing, cutting-edge data and analysis, and a relentless focus on delivering meaningful results. Under this new model, we are also engaging with the world's brightest problem-solvers to bend the curve of progress. Over the past five years, we have launched five *Grand Challenges for Development* grant competitions to source, test, and scale groundbreaking ideas.

Now in its fourth round, *Saving Lives at Birth: A Grand Challenge for Development* is aimed at developing technologies that can save the lives of mothers and children during the most vulnerable hours around the time of birth. After 2,000 innovative proposals from 102 countries and more than 60 winners, a constellation of lifesaving innovations now stretches from the United States to India to Uganda.

For example, students at Rice University developed an easy-to-use, battery-operated bubble CPAP machine that resuscitates newborns and costs just a fraction of the price of existing equipment. In early tests, the bubble CPAP *tripled* newborn survival rates.

In Nepal, chlorhexidine, an antiseptic gel that mothers can apply to an infant's umbilical cord stump, is preventing deadly infections and cutting infant mortality by nearly 23%. Today, a local Nepali pharmaceutical company is helping deliver chlorhexidine free of charge to expectant mothers across the country, and efforts are underway to introduce it in 15 additional countries.

We are proud of our progress, but more must be done. From universities to refugee camps, we have seen that ingenuity and good ideas are universal. To end preventable child death, we must continue to have our eye on the future—by unifying and accelerating the efforts of the leaders, partners, and innovators who will shape it.

Rajiv Shah is the Administrator of the US Agency for International Development and former Chief Scientist of the US Department of Agriculture.

Chapter 88

Transformative Leadership

KENJI SHIBUYA

At a time when the global health community faces so much uncertainty, we need transformative leaders to dream and ask "why not?"

In 1994, I bumped into Marie-Louise on a street in a huge Rwandan refugee camp in Goma, Zaire, where I worked as a medical officer for a Japanese NGO. She had arrived there after walking day and night over hundreds of miles from Kigali to escape one of the worst genocides in human history. In her arms she held her two children, who were malnourished and dying from shigella. Luckily I was able to help her, and a standard antibiotics treatment saved their lives. In return, Marie-Louise offered to help around our clinic in the camp. She was a schoolteacher and initially I did not expect much as she did not have any medical background. But I was completely wrong—she changed our activities with her leadership. She was instrumental in bringing in the best possible resources from the camp, including nurses, dentists, security guards, and drivers, and she worked tirelessly on medical outreach to the refugees. She was indispensable to the first ever peacekeeping operation by the Japanese Self-Defense Force. During a time of war, disease, and brutality, she brought us hope for the future—much like the person described in The Pretenders' song "Show Me":

> You, with your innocence and grace
> Restore some pride and dignity
> To a world in decline

Two decades later, I visited Rwanda once again at Marie-Louise's invitation, and found a nation where everything had changed. Women and children were safely walking the streets at night. The Hutus and Tutsis had succeeded in unity and reconciliation, and the country had achieved stability and security. Agnes Binagwaho, Rwanda's Minister of Health, invited us to breakfast under the palm trees and shared her vision for addressing the new challenges to her country's health system. Surely many issues remain and new hurdles lie ahead, but the approximately 70% reduction in under-5 mortality in Rwanda between 2000 and 2012 is one of the most successful stories in global health today. This remarkable turnaround is not only due to political stability and rapid economic growth, but can also be attributed to the implementation of essential intervention packages with a focus on health equity, including women and the disabled, under the visionary leadership of Agnes and her colleagues.

These two women were born in the same country with radically different destinies and responsibilities, but they have one thing in common: both of them are transformative leaders who have saved lives. President John F. Kennedy once said, "The problems of the world cannot possibly be solved by skeptics or cynics, whose horizons are limited by the obvious realities. We need men [and women] who can dream of things that never were and ask, why not?"

Transformative leaders are not just professionals, but can come from any walk of life and can be found in even the most difficult of circumstances. They see the world as it should be, challenge the status quo, and make a difference in people's lives. In health, especially, simple and cost-effective technologies, such as vaccination and family planning, maternal education, or tobacco control can solve many of the biggest problems the global health community faces. More resources have become available to address these challenges. Yet, we still see many maternal and child deaths, resurgent and emergent communicable diseases, and a growing epidemic of noncommunicable diseases. Technology or money is one thing, but what matters most in solving these problems are transformative leaders who can achieve their goals even when resources are limited.

The world is becoming increasingly interconnected and interdependent. Health systems, both domestic and global, cannot escape the consequences of globalization, nor can they ignore its benefits—not only diseases, but also doctors, nurses, and patients move across countries. Population health has continued to improve in leaps and bounds over the past century.

However, globalization has not succeeded in ensuring that everyone has access to basic health services. Health systems are polarized in many countries, especially those under transition, with quality private care for the rich and meager public services for the rest. Wars, brutality, and inequity still stand in the way of progress. At a time when the global health community faces huge financial, political, and organizational uncertainty, we need transformative leaders at the community, national, and global levels, like these two Rwandan women who asked, "why not?"

Kenji Shibuya is Professor of Global Health Policy at the University of Tokyo and former Coordinator with the World Health Organization.

Chapter 89

Global Health Citizenship

MICHEL SIDIBÉ

Our increasingly interdependent world demands a collective cognitive shift to global health citizenship, wherein empowered people claim their rights and take responsibility for their health and that of fellow citizens.

Albert Einstein provocatively argued that "the world as we have created it is a process of our thinking. It cannot be changed without changing our thinking."

The one change most needed to transform global health is neither a magic bullet drug, nor a shiny new institution. It is a global collective shift in consciousness. We have created a globalizing world that is both hyperconnected and interdependent. And yet, we continue to assume that the main responsibility for people's health lies with nation states. While countries continue to perform critical roles, today's global health challenges demand collaborative multi-sectoral action by governments, civil society, and the private sector that cannot be performed by any government alone. Building on Julio Frenk's conceptualization of "global solidarity" in the context of a "global society," I argue that robust accountability can only be ensured, and individual and collective responsibility for health upheld, by instigating a profound shift in our mindset toward *global health citizenship*.

The world will continue to change beyond our recognition. The rapid explosion of chronic progressive diseases demonstrates how fast the global health landscape can change. These illnesses also shine light on the complex interlinkages of public health with political, economic, social, and cultural determinants of health, including the impact of the tobacco, food, alcohol, and other industries. The global HIV/AIDS pandemic was the first to reveal the implications of an interconnected world. Air travel among global hubs for transnational flows of goods, money, and people meant that the HIV virus spread globally before anyone even realized it existed. Simultaneously, the response underscored the need for global collective action and the power of emerging forms of global solidarity and citizenship in confronting global challenges

Furthermore, HIV/AIDS has demonstrated that the twentieth century paradigm of development—where one part of the world has money and the other part of the world has problems—is obsolete. It was set up decades ago to respond to a set of problems defined during a period in which we no longer live; it is unfit to address emerging health threats and needs. We must shift from charity to sustainability. Global solidarity combined with shared responsibility is the only viable alternative.

And with it must come a new *global health citizen*—a political citizen who claims rights, duties, responsibilities, and membership in a political community. In this community, each individual is empowered to claim their rights to health and to demand action and answers from decision-makers. Yet membership is not guaranteed without an accompanying responsibility for the health of fellow members of society. We must grasp the opportunity presented by the post-2015 development agenda to agree on a framework with the global health citizen at its center, as defined by three core elements.

First, global health citizenship is about people-centered activism. It is about forcing a shift from "beneficiaries" and "consumers" to active change agents. To reflect this, the planning model is transformed from a top-down approach to one driven by people—what I call the democratization of problem-solving. HIV/AIDS shows this is possible. In the early days of the epidemic, people living with HIV/AIDS, refusing indignity and injustice, came together to demand change from governments and the private sector alike. They organized themselves and their communities. They led a paradigm shift from disease- to people-centered approaches, and they championed socially participatory decision-making. We need more of this sort of democratization for people at the margins—including women, young people, and the bottom billion living in middle-income countries.

Second, global health citizenship is about ensuring modernized accountability mechanisms and governance systems that leverage interconnectedness and are fit for an interdependent world. Through their hyperconnectivity, change agents can collaborate to hold service providers and decision-makers accountable. In Kenya, the Ushahidi Platform demonstrates the potential of harnessing technology to successfully create virtual world networks for this purpose. Originally used to map incidents of violence and peace efforts throughout the country, this platform has developed into an online information sharing hub which empowers citizens to hold governments to account.

Third, and most crucially, global health citizenship is about the citizen taking responsibility for their health and the health of others. This requires a new social contract for health. In many middle-income countries, we see threats to citizenship posed by growing inequality and the aspirations of the middle classes when the prospect of wealth blinds them from obligations to other members of their society. We need not only new global *health* citizens but global citizens who take individual and collective responsibility for the well-being and sustainable future of both people and planet.

Ultimately, sustainable development requires a rethink of citizenship. While I call for citizen activism, citizen accountability, and citizen compacts, I am guided by Mahatma Gandhi: "The spirit of democracy cannot be imposed from without. It has to come from within."

Michel Sidibé is Executive Director of the Joint United Nations Programme on HIV/AIDS (UNAIDS) and Under-Secretary-General of the United Nations.

Chapter 90

Harmonizing Health

AKINWANDE OLUWOLE "WOLE" SOYINKA

Amid endless scientific advances, an openness to new approaches—even conflicting ones—is imperative.

Any statement on the relevance of traditional or cultural findings to modern curative practices should never be viewed as an invitation to replace the latter with the former, but as a complement to the world's advances in the medical sciences. In proposing this as a "transformative insight," my intent is no more than a reorientation of the contemporary physician mind. It does, however, implicate a drastic transformation of today's overall medical outlook, including its physical structures. Since these form a part of our environment, they affect both the tempo of healing and the body's response to treatment. Nothing new, just the ancient "harmonization of the universe of the human body and mind to the external universe." From the Native Americans to the *sangoma* of South Africa, from the *babalawo* of the Yoruba to the currently fashionable Chinese traditional medicine, this harmonization has remained the basis of medical science until the near total separation of body, mind, and culture in modern medicine.

The Western world remains manifestly—and justifiably—proud of a heritage that values the anatomization of the human body and advances in its chemical intervention. However, we have become detached from the more holistic, though seemingly "unscientific" origins that are now largely viewed through the distorting prism of superstitious beliefs. I believe, however—and this is no prediction but the fruit of observation—that there will be an increasing reversion to the early holism in responding to today's health needs. This is already evident even in many parts of the Western world. More than the actual treatment, the ambiance of powders, unguents, herbs, barks, potions, and the like impart a greater sense of closeness to Nature's curative resources than those gleaming, deodorized, and impersonal clinics that also exclude the patient from participation in his or her own healing process. Being permitted to view X-rays, C-scans, or even womb motions for the pregnant admittedly indicates changes in attitude. Such "inclusiveness" indicates some advance (more accurately, return) to the participatory role of the patient as it often exists in, for example, the *babalawo* of the Yoruba. As the world of medicine grows increasingly enlightened, however, future generations may look forward to the most ultramodern teaching hospitals actually offering consultation rooms where patients can look into the traditional clinic of the *sangoma* or *shaman* for a role in an integrated healing system.

Does this pose a danger of duplication in the patient's regimen? Well, even in Western hospitals, patients are still required to complete a form stating what prescriptions—including "nature supplements"—they are currently taking. Would another line be added for the disclosure of nonmaterial prescriptions, such as invocations or incantations? No, not any more than today's religious patient chants "Praise the Lord" or intones "Allahu Akbar" before swallowing his or her daily prescription. What matters is the near certainty of a heightened sensibility through participation of culture-derived processes, and a greater understanding of the interior language of the body's universe, assisting the Western-trained physicians in their own diagnoses and prescriptions.

My favorite example of this practical collaboration is the story of Jacob. It is one that is current, globally acknowledged, and to whose results I can personally testify. His healing odyssey began in California and ended in a spinal injury clinic just outside Accra, Ghana, headed by a Ghanaian doctor trained in the Western tradition.

Jacob's agony was not a sight for weak stomachs. It was a case that stumped even the most specialized American hospitals like the Cedar

Sinai in Los Angeles, which finally gave up and downgraded his treatment to extreme pain management.

It was at this point that Jacob sought treatment in Ghana. At the Ghanaian clinic, his condition was immediately recognized. The doctor tossed his medications—all 19 of them—into the rubbish bin, and followed a process that was based on the application of a poultice made from local herbal leaves. The harvesting of those leaves was a ritual scrupulously retained by the clinic. The season, the time of day, the procession into the forest, the solemn chants were all ritualistically followed as they have been from a time no one can precisely recall. Jacob's treatment lasted three weeks.

Back in California, I was busy in my study when a man I failed to recognize entered, grinning. As I continued to stare, he broke into a Ghanaian dance—the *kpalongo*! Jacob? Why indeed it was the same Jacob, who for nearly three years had been wheelchair-bound!

Jacob's transformation is a testament to the healing powers that lie in the harmonization of the universe of the body with the external universe. Was it not on this holistic path that our earliest healers first set their feet? I cannot help proposing that the future of healing lies in that past, in its selective adaptation.

Wole Soyinka is a Nigerian playwright and political activist who received the Nobel Prize for Literature in 1986.

Chapter 91

Public Health 2.0

JONAS GAHR STØRE

Upgrading public health policy is needed to tackle noncommunicable diseases and represents the most sensible decision for policymakers in the twenty-first century.

A modern public health policy stands as the strongest strategic option for national health systems in the twenty-first century. Policymakers and health professionals will be faced with many hard choices as the technological revolution in health moves forward within a context of budgetary restraints.

We need to reinvent public health as the defining influencer of contemporary policymaking. Whether it's implementing effective measures for prevention of disease or creating a framework for universal maternal and child health, policy has the ability to positively address the social health determinants that lead to our world's systemic inequities.

When I served as Norway's Minister of Health, I recall a meeting with my counterpart from Malawi. She had still pressing priorities to deal with linked to communicable diseases such as HIV, tuberculosis, and malaria. But most of our conversation dealt with how the health service in both our countries, Norway and Malawi, could develop meaningful policies of prevention to halt the tide of noncommunicable and lifestyle diseases. We easily agreed on the obvious: that prevention is far more effective than cure, particularly in that states can avoid huge budgets strains from expensive treatment and care. This discussion is what led me to conceive of my model for Public Health 2.0, alluding to the need to upgrade how we think about public health and how we connect the various components of a modern public health policy.

I presented to the Norwegian Parliament a white paper on public health policy as a key tool to combat the rise in noncommunicable diseases. As I worked on that paper I came across some valuable lessons from the past. Norway's transition to a welfare state—a structure in which citizens' health and the meeting of their social needs are subsidized by government—was greatly enhanced from the outset by a comprehensive effort to introduce public health policies and structural policies that allowed Norwegians from all walks of life to make wiser choices regarding health.

As Norway entered the twentieth century, its persisting poverty was evident in its glut of early deaths from tuberculosis—a disease known to prey on those on the poorer end of the socioeconomic spectrum. Across Norway, as with most nations, the key risk factor to ill health was poverty. I read from history that on the list of demands from the emerging labor movement were public health issues: clean water, safe housing, universal health coverage, better child health services. In short, a long list of public health policies to be implemented in a way that would reach all, universal measures that would not distinguish between rich and poor, structural policies that would influence individual behavior. These policies were largely successful, and public health policy advances underpinned the transition of Norway in becoming an advanced welfare state with core health and care services available to all, either free of charge or at a low cost.

Today's risk factors emerge from our personal choices as constrained by the environment to construct our lifestyle: what we eat and drink, how we exercise, how we travel. Designing policies to address the health challenges associated with lifestyle will require nothing less than a broad mobilization that both arms the public with the information they need to make informed choices and implements policies that make such choices easy in our communities.

Public policy at all levels is plagued by the organization of policy areas into silos: economics, health, education, welfare, culture, and so on. A first step in integration is to see public health policy areas in a much more common context. On the basis of international targets as set out by the world's states, we need national strategies that connect policies from all sectors, including government, business, and civil society.

Public health policy will be the key to dealing with the emerging noncommunicable disease epidemic. Democracies are in a strong position because effective public health requires involvement, ownership, and participation—the fundamental tenets of democratic government. They can take a lead in developing Public Health 2.0 to address the growing, daunting health challenges facing us.

Governmental systems offer great potential for integration and advancement of public health and prevention. To take one example: modern public transportation systems can be developed to integrate both public health targets and environmental concerns, both to help limit injuries from traffic accidents and to help limit emissions that cause respiratory diseases.

Public Health 2.0 is about streamlining, integrating, and upgrading, and it is the most important and sensible thing policymakers could opt for in the twenty-first century.

Jonas Gahr Støre is Leader of the Norwegian Labour Party, Member of the Norwegian Storting, and former Minister of Foreign Affairs and Minister of Health of Norway.

Chapter 92

Tax Reform

DAVID STUCKLER

Global health interventions require funding, but where is it going to come from?

Global health policy has, to its detriment, gone through a series of faddish, silver-bullet ideas to solve its problems. One week mass circumcision to tackle HIV/AIDS might be in vogue. The next week it's a mosquito zapper to stop malaria. Put simply, there is no panacea to the world's biggest pandemics. Tackling avoidable deaths from HIV/AIDS, heart disease, obesity, tuberculosis, alcohol poisoning, and suicide, to name a few, will take commitment, time, energy, and, importantly, resources. The sooner we recognize this, the better.

What we can do is put in place the building blocks of robust health and social protection systems. There is an emerging consensus of the importance of guaranteeing a base level of support for all. Margaret Chan, Director-General of the World Health Organization, says that "universal health coverage is one the most powerful concepts that WHO has to offer." Similarly, the International Labour Organization has repeatedly called for establishing a social protection floor. The global commitment to providing antiretrovirals for all persons who live with HIV/AIDS, alongside the development of pandemic preparedness measures, are among the first important steps to establishing global protection systems.

But to make all this possible, global tax reform is desperately needed. People don't often think about taxes as a global health issue, yet it's the single most important way of ensuring that resource-deprived countries can finance stable infrastructure, programs, and services that promote health.

The importance of taxes to global health is evident from even a cursory look at cross-national data (Fig. 92.1). Research shows that those societies which harvest greater tax resources tend to have substantially higher levels of government health spending. This pattern holds even after adjusting for a country's GDP per capita and, when taxes factor into the model, the commonly seen relationship of economic development and public health spending disappears.

Unsurprisingly, the additional health resources associated with tax revenues correspond to greater numbers of doctors, nurses, and community health workers per capita, higher access to skilled birth attendants per capita, narrower inequalities in access to immunizations, and, overall, better health for women and children.

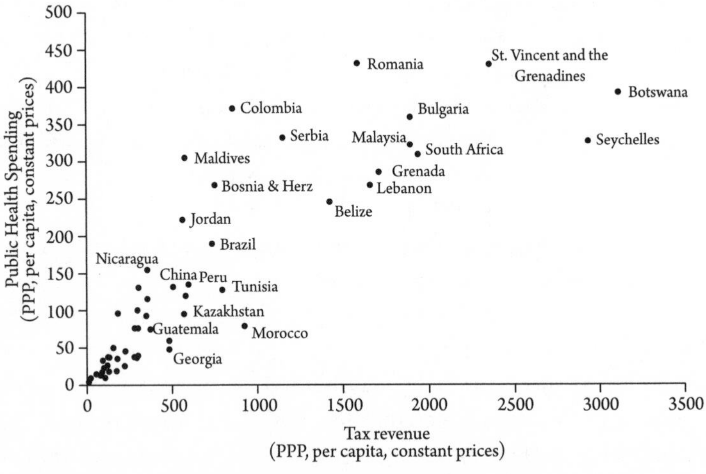

Figure 92.1 Governments that harvest greater tax resources tend to spend more on health. Tax revenue and public health spending are adjusted for inflation and purchasing power parity (PPP). From World Bank, World Development Indicators, 2014 edition.

The implication is clear. When more financial resources enter into a democratic commons, they tend to flow toward greater health investments.

Take India, for example. Despite its remarkable economic growth, its public health system is emaciated. The Indian government spends about $28 per person per year, ranking it at about 172nd in the world. This stems, in large part, from relatively low tax intake. The country's effective tax rate is 10.4% of GDP. If India were to increase its tax revenue to the proportion of GDP seen in high-income countries (about 14.4%), it would generate an additional revenue of $44.30 USD per person. This increase in funds alone would be sufficient to achieve universal health care in India at the estimated cost of $24 USD per person annually.

There is an important nuance to this call for increasing taxes. It matters how we raise the tax revenues. In the majority of low-income countries, tax systems are highly regressive. They rely on consumption and sales-based tax regimes, rather than taxing capital gains and firms. It is commonly debated whether doing the latter would harm economic growth. Irrespective of this debate, it is clear that these regressive taxes do correlate significantly with worse child survival and maternal mortality rates.

Generating political support for global tax reform is a critical challenge for everyone. Increasing taxes is often unpopular. Fiscal conservatives are especially likely to oppose this plan. They strongly oppose tax increases in high-income countries. CEOs of multinational corporations and powerful investment banks are equally vocal against the prospect of tax increases in developing economies, where they look to lower the costs of their labor supply.

Over the past four decades, these elites have pushed a so-called 'neoliberal' model of economic development that emphasizes low taxes, weak unions, and small government. This fiscal conservativism was embedded in debt conditionalities of international financial institutions including the International Monetary Fund and World Bank. In this macroeconomic context, economic growth alone will not be sufficient to build health systems without a corresponding increase in tax revenues. Nor will increasing donor-aid resources help low-tax countries become truly independent.

Central to making the case for increasing taxes would be demonstrating to the public that these tax dollars will indeed translate into meaningful benefits. We also need to know more about improving the effectiveness of tax systems and closing international tax havens and loopholes. With the growing intensity of debate about inequality, the rise of the top 1%, and tax reform in high-income countries, should we not also extend our view to the global picture?

The task for those of us working in global health policy is to help make the seemingly impossible a reality within our time. Tax reform is a good place to start.

David Stuckler is a Professor of Political Economy and Sociology and Fellow of Christ Church at the University of Oxford.

Chapter 93

Investing in a Grand Convergence

LARRY SUMMERS

If we can increase our health sector investments to make powerful vaccines, medicines, and other health tools available to everyone, we could achieve a "grand convergence" in global health within our lifetimes.

A once-in-human-history opportunity to transform global health is presently at our fingertips. About 200 years ago, life expectancy was short and child and maternal mortality rates were high in all countries around the world. This was the universal human condition. But then, beginning in the early part of the eighteenth century, the world experienced a great divergence: rich countries saw their rates of mortality plummet, thanks in large part to advances in public health and medicine, while poor countries were left behind.

But now we are on the cusp of a remarkable achievement. If we can increase our health sector investments to make powerful vaccines, medicines, and other health tools available to everyone, we could achieve a "grand convergence" in global health within our lifetimes.

Within just one generation we could reduce the rates of infectious, maternal, and child deaths in nearly all low- and middle-income countries to the low levels seen today in wealthier parts of the world (Fig. 93.1).

Currently an astonishing 1 in 10 children in poor countries die before their fifth birthday; by 2035, we could reduce that death rate

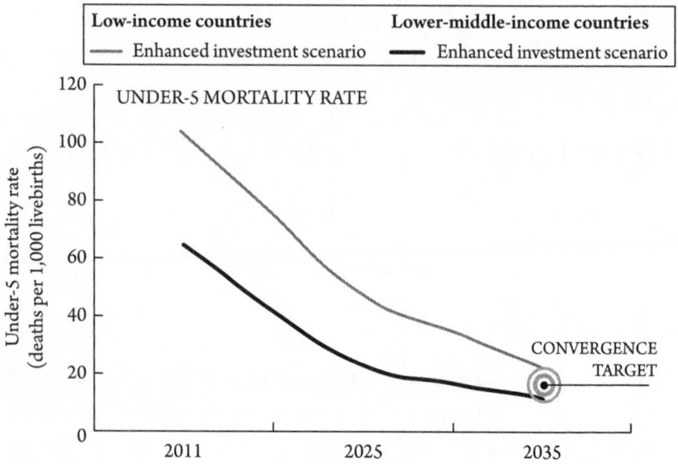

Figure 93.1 Estimated decline in child mortality rates from enhanced health sector investments. The "convergence target" is 20 deaths per 1,000 live births, similar to the current child mortality rate in high-performing middle-income countries.

down to 1 in 50. We could prevent 10 million maternal, child, and adult deaths each year from 2035 onwards.

Collectively, across all countries, we have the financial and the ever-improving technological capabilities to achieve this grand convergence. The ambitious, yet feasible, roadmap for making that happen has three key components.

First, we must mobilize financing for health. The price tag for low- and lower-middle-income countries to achieve convergence will be an additional $70 billion per year from now to 2035. The good news is that these countries are on course to add $10 trillion per year to the size of their economies in that same period. In other words, public investment of less than 1% of this GDP growth could fund the grand convergence. Taxing harmful substances like tobacco, alcohol, and sugar-sweetened sodas, plus removing public subsidies on fossil fuels, could also mobilize domestic funding to support convergence, while helping to curb noncommunicable diseases such as heart disease and cancers.

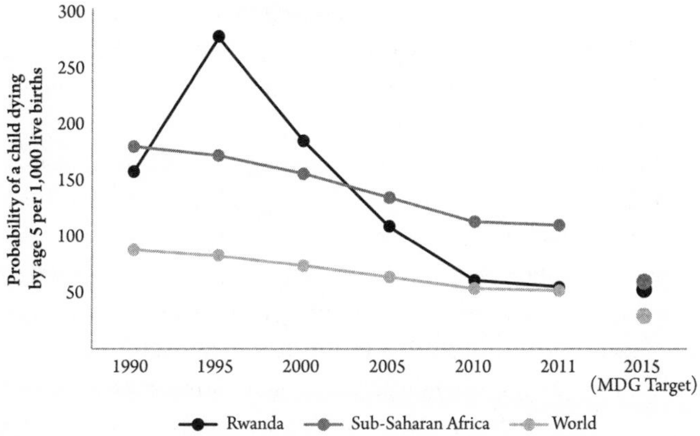

Figure 93.2 Rapid decline in child mortality in Rwanda, 1995–2011.
From Paul Farmer, et al. *BMJ 346 (2013)*: f65.

Second, we must invest in the most cost-effective health interventions. Maternal and child deaths, and deaths from infections, can be rapidly and dramatically reduced by a highly focused effort to ensure that everyone has access to the most cost-effective health tools and services. Rwanda has shown the way, recently achieving the fastest fall in child deaths in recorded history (Fig. 93.2), from 275 deaths per 1,000 live births in 1995 to 54 per 1,000 live births by 2011. There is nothing mysterious about the "Rwanda miracle," as it has come to be known—child deaths were slashed by boosting rates of vaccinations and preventing and treating major childhood killers like malaria, pneumonia, and diarrhea. Replicating the same approach in other countries would replicate the same results.

Third, we must fund avenues of global public good, like research and development (R&D) and the management of cross-border threats. A grand convergence cannot be achieved with today's tools alone. We will need new health technologies to fully close the health equity gap.

The most important way in which the international community can support the grand convergence is by funding the discovery, development, and delivery of the next generation of medicines, vaccines, diagnostics, and devices. International funding for R&D targeted at diseases that disproportionately affect poor countries must be doubled from current levels—to $6 billion USD per year by 2020, with half the increment coming from upper middle-income countries like China, India, and South Africa.

We must also get serious about tackling cross-border threats, like antibiotic resistance, counterfeit medicines, and flu pandemics. The next flu pandemic could be far deadlier than the 1918 epidemic that killed more than 50 million people in an era before mass, international transit.

One of the most profound and striking benefits of achieving a grand convergence is that, in addition to the vast public health gains, there would also be a huge economic payoff from investing in its achievement. Every dollar invested from 2015 to 2035 would return between 9 and 20 dollars. This is an astonishing return on investment.

Investing in the grand convergence represents the greatest opportunity available on the planet to improve human welfare. No other possible investment comes even close.

Lawrence H. Summers is President Emeritus and Charles W. Eliot University Professor of Harvard University and a former US Treasury Secretary.

Chapter 94

Health in a Multipolar World

KEIZO TAKEMI

Human security should be an overarching governor of our future health interventions.

As a politician, I am an admirer of Abraham Lincoln. His words, "Determine that the thing can and shall be done, and then we shall find the way," are relevant to global health today.

The first decade of the twenty-first century will go down in history as a golden era for global health, when financing increased enormously and the Millennium Development Goals provided a global framework for investments to mitigate the vicious circle of poverty and ill health. Past achievements in health goals were possible because of massive investment through new financial mechanisms and numerous partnerships with civil society, foundations, and other private entities including industry. Governments no longer have a monopoly on health, as a more inclusive approach has been adopted.

At the same time, the geopolitical and economic landscapes of countries are rapidly changing. China has become the second largest economy, new economies have emerged, and American power has relatively declined. As such it has become difficult to govern the world with unipolar theory wherein one state holds most of the economic and military influence. We are now beginning to evolve into a multipolar world in terms of geopolitics as well as global health. The new paradigm requires transformations in thinking and approaches to governing the partnerships among various stakeholders in global health and redefining the division of responsibilities for global public goods among states with consideration of the changing power balance.

There have been lengthy and complicated consultations among various stakeholders about the future of international development, which reveals that we are in a transitional phase of global governance. We do not know the exact goals that will be agreed on for the post-2015 agenda; however, in my view, human security should carry significant weight. Human security aims to promote three freedoms—freedom from want, freedom from fear, and freedom to live in dignity in a comprehensive manner. It also requires synergy between protection and empowerment of the most vulnerable populations at all levels—community, national, and global—while emphasizing the community as the target unit for designing policies and using them to make real changes in people's lives.

Japan has promoted human security through its policies related to the United Nations and official development assistance. In 1998, Prime Minister Keizo Obuchi proposed human security as a key concept for Japan's new resilient pacifism, and prioritized health as instrumental to achieving human security at the G8 Summits in Okinawa and Toyako. Last year, Prime Minister Shinzo Abe announced his commitment to promoting universal health coverage globally and making it Japan's flagship commitment to global health. Universal health coverage encompasses "universalism and equity" instead of common goals among various stakeholders regardless of the diseases being targeted, communicable or noncommunicable. It enables each country to explore its own path to sustainably responding to the real needs of their most vulnerable populations. Universal health coverage, therefore, indicates the priority that Japan accords to human security.

To create sustainable and equitable global governance in health, Japan, together with the global community, should recommit to human security and to solving global challenges beyond its borders by helping people live healthy, productive, and dignified lives.

First, we need to strengthen human resources for health at the community, national, and global levels in the public sector, academia, and the private sector (including business and civil society). We need people who are able to develop and implement policy in order to achieve better health and well-being for the most vulnerable people in each country's unique context. Though the roles and responsibilities of each sector differ at each level, practical policy-oriented and solution-oriented minds are required.

Second, we need to find better ways to govern partnerships among states, civil society, foundations, and other private entities. The current multipolar environment has challenged the governance of international organizations such as the World Health Organization and the World Bank. The governance structure of the Global Fund to Fight AIDS, Tuberculosis, and Malaria may be a good example for exploring global governance in the future because of its requirement for nongovernmental actors to be fully engaged in decisions at headquarters as well as in each partner country, but further explorations are needed.

I believe it is critical for all of us to continue committing to health alongside other global challenges. I hope we will follow Lincoln's advice and find a way to do the things that we determine should be done.

Keizo Takemi is a Member of Japan's House of Councillors and former Senior Vice-Minister of Health, Labour, and Welfare of Japan.

Chapter 95

Midwives Save Women's Lives

CHRISTY TURLINGTON BURNS

Advancing midwifery care around the world will help entire families, communities, and countries achieve better health for all.

The statistics speak volumes: More than a third of all births take place without a midwife or other skilled health-care provider in attendance. Only one in three women living in rural areas of developing countries receive adequate prenatal care. An increase in the number of trained midwives would save the lives of hundreds of thousands of women each year and improve the health and well-being of millions more who suffer debilitating, life-altering injuries during childbirth. Scaling-up midwifery would enhance the physical health and economic security of every woman, her children, and her grandchildren. Without question, increasing the numbers of trained midwives would have an immediate, positive, and dramatic effect on global health.

Yet we face a global shortage of midwives. Every day, about 800 women die because they do not have access to trained midwives or other skilled health-care providers or because there are no well-staffed, well-supplied health-care facilities nearby. New research has shown that if we scaled up the number of skilled midwives in the world, we could reduce maternal mortality by two-thirds. That's because midwives can provide quality care and support for a woman during her entire reproductive life. They not only assist in childbirth, but they provide critical prenatal and postnatal care. Midwives are arguably the best option to handle most straightforward deliveries, especially in low-resource settings where obstetricians and other specially trained physicians are scarce.

So why aren't there more midwives available to meet this pressing need? One reason is that training to be a midwife can be expensive. Many prospective students find the costs prohibitive. In addition, hospitals and training centers often impose strict limits on the number of students they will accept into a training program in order to keep their own costs down. Further, once a student is accepted and graduates from a program, she is often poorly compensated for her skills, a fact that may dissuade others from taking on the expense of midwifery training.

Another reason why there aren't more midwives practicing around the world is that, in some areas, the term "midwife" continues to carry a negative connotation. Midwives are often viewed as less capable than physicians. In truth, well-trained midwives provide high-quality health services and are crucial for providing the continuum of health care that all women need. A qualified midwife can guide a woman not only through pregnancy, labor, birth and the post-partum period, but she can also assist with the care of a newborn, reinforce breastfeeding, assist in post-partum recovery and subsequent birth planning and spacing. Midwives are also essential for identifying high-risk situations and determining when a mother needs more specialized care.

A third reason why there aren't enough midwives to meet our current and future needs is that midwifery is a difficult job, and those difficulties increase exponentially in areas of severe poverty that lack basic support, medical supplies, and adequate infrastructure. It's no coincidence that these are the very areas where midwives are most needed. Once trained, many midwives choose to practice in urban areas where there is more support available. While understandable, it leaves women in the most impoverished areas without access to proper care.

Thankfully, there are at least three tangible steps we can take to ensure that we train a greater number of midwives to meet the urgent global demand. First, we need to provide more opportunities for training, including scholarships for midwifery students to attend school. Second, we must integrate midwives into existing medical and social structures. And third, we should incentivize midwives to work in rural areas by providing stipends and ensuring they have necessary medical supplies.

Quality maternal and reproductive health care is every woman's right; but women continue to die at a rate of one every two minutes while giving birth. We know the solution to this crisis. Consistent evidence-based health care for the world's mothers will save their lives, and midwifery is an essential part of that care. Only when health-care advocates demand better care for women and make that demand a global priority will we see improvement in the lives of women and the health and welfare of generations to come.

Christy Turlington Burns is Founder of Every Mother Counts.

Chapter 96

Smart Data

KENT WALKER

The Information Revolution is transforming the future of public health.

The numbers are breathtaking. While it took us 150 years between 1750 and 1900 to double our store of information, today we double the amount of stored information every year. We have created 90% of the world's data in the last two years alone.

The Information Revolution is now empowering patients, distributing knowledge, and saving lives. These advances are not only transforming health-care research but also democratizing the nature of medicine.

It starts with the technology of information: the costs of storing, processing, and transmitting data are all asymptotically approaching zero. What used to be hard and expensive is becoming easy and almost free, unlocking remarkable possibilities.

Five years ago, sequencing one's genome required mortgaging one's home—now we can charge the expense to our credit cards. Falling costs make new treatments accessible to millions.

But the real magic lies not in big numbers or even lower costs, but in new insights. Data alone isn't interesting. Data is to knowledge what sand is to silicon chips. But hidden among the infinite potential correlations lie the profound causal links that will help us diagnose and cure disease. It's the analysis and understanding of these links that make the difference. Instead of "Big Data," think "Smart Data."

Smart Data is powerful. Genetics revolutionizes cancer treatment by giving us a deeper understanding of disease variants. For example, a drug against melanoma that's 2% effective is essentially worthless. But if we can distinguish 50 different types of melanoma, each 2% of the whole, a drug might be 100% effective against one of those types. Suddenly, we've found a miracle cure for a rarer disease. When we look more closely, "rare diseases" become commonplace, and the dream of personalized medicine comes true.

Physiology can be even more important than genetics. Our well-being—our "health output"—depends on many inputs: genomes, epigenetics, diets, activity, environments, and microbiomes. Yet we lack a sophisticated approach to measuring health inputs or outputs, making it harder to tune inputs for better results. Now that's changing. New wearable devices track fitness, steps, diet, and sleep. And that's just the beginning. The OECD is developing data maps of dementia, which are products of a "multi-factorial" effort combining heterogeneous behavioral, genetic, environmental, and clinical data sets. Doctors are using social networks to develop disease prevention registries. And consumers are crowdsourcing medicine, demanding increased access to information, and using novel platforms to build powerful knowledge networks among those most motivated to find and share information.

Smart Data can also benefit entire communities. Researchers can analyze not just raw patterns of disease, but also online signals like search queries, tweets, and social media posts to predict outbreaks, anticipate humanitarian disasters, and coordinate lifesaving development work.

Of course, while medicine's Hippocratic oath emphasizes avoiding harm, Silicon Valley's "launch and iterate" spirit promotes widespread and dramatic progress. Technology streamlines systems, cuts costs, and increases consumer choice. But how should public health balance consumer protection and empowerment?

Information about your own risk factors empowers you as a health-care consumer, letting you make smarter choices and contribute to your own care. Unfortunately some people can be misled or use information to make bad choices. But that doesn't mean we must ban horoscopes or junk diets entirely. We should instead promote Smart Data education, and work toward raising everyone's level of knowledge. Trained professionals can help interpret data, counseling patients before they take action and providing advice to whole communities.

A second set of questions involve ownership and use of data. Markets have helped improve social welfare across cultures and centuries—a globalized world economy lifted hundreds of millions of people from extreme poverty. Yet health-care markets continue to face concerns over self-interested actions and misaligned incentives. We have seen debates over the ownership of genes and genetic tools (as in the "Hela" gene strain or the *Myriad* patent case) as well as the collateral learning from health data. We need rules that foster both the freedom and the incentive to innovate.

Privacy poses a third set of issues. Medical research has traditionally relied on anonymized data to protect privacy. This is harder in the world of genetics. Even there, injecting "noise" into data sets can address concerns about re-identification, and informed consent can let people knowingly contribute to research. Still, consent can be tricky, especially for evolving technologies. How do people consent to uses that we haven't imagined yet? We need to respect individual choice, while recognizing the collective benefits of sharing health data. And we need to forge a social consensus on data research, information exchange, and the sensitivity of different types of data.

Public policy can help us find solutions, but not without creative contributions from a range of participants. Regulation should focus on the potential misuses of information, weighing the benefits and risks of new research. But let's not lose sight of the remarkable potential of Smart Data to provide a data-driven and people-centric future for global health.

Kent Walker is Senior Vice President and General Counsel of Google Inc.

BOOKS RECOMMENDED BY CONTRIBUTORS

Acemoglu, Daron, and James Robinson. 2012. *Why Nations Fail: The Origins of Power, Prosperity, and Poverty*. New York: Crown Business.

Achebe, Chinua. 1995. *Things Fall Apart: A Novel*. New York: Fawcett Crest Books.

Barrett, Scott. 2010. *Why Cooperate? The Incentive to Supply Global Public Goods*. New York: Oxford University Press.

Barry, John M. 2004. *The Great Influenza: The Story of the Deadliest Pandemic in History*. London: Penguin Books.

Behrman, Greg. 2009. *The Invisible People: How the U.S. Has Slept Through the Global AIDS Pandemic, the Greatest Humanitarian Catastrophe of Our Time*. New York: Free Press.

Boo, Katherine. 2012. *Behind the Beautiful Forevers: Life, Death, and Hope in a Mumbai Undercity*. New York: Random House.

Brown, Lester R. 2010. *World on the Edge*. New York: W. W. Norton.

Brown, Tim. 2009. *Change By Design: How Design Thinking Transforms Organizations and Inspires Innovation*. New York: Harper Business.

Brynjolfsson, Erik, and Andrew McAfee. 2014. *The Second Machine Age: Work, Progress, and Prosperity in a Time of Brilliant Technologies*. New York: W. W. Norton.

Clinton, Hillary Rodham. 2014. *Hard Choices*. New York: Simon & Schuster.

Cohen, Jessica, and William Easterly, eds. 2009. *What Works in Development? Thinking Big and Thinking Small*. Washington DC: Brookings Institution Press.

Collier, Paul. 2008. *The Bottom Billion: Why the Poorest Countries are Failing and What Can be Done About It*. Oxford: Oxford University Press.

Coulter, Angela. 2011. *Engaging Patients in Healthcare*. New York: Open University Press.

Crisp, Nigel. 2010. *Turning the World Upside Down: The Search for Global Health in the 21st Century*. London: CRC Press.

Crosby, Alfred W. 1990. *America's Forgotten Pandemic: The Influenza of 1918*. Cambridge, UK: Cambridge University Press.

Daar, Abdallah, and Peter A. Singer. 2011. *The Grandest Challenge: Taking Life-Saving Science from Lab to Village*. Toronto: Doubleday Canada.

Davies, Sally, Jonathan Grant, and Mike Catchpole. 2014. *The Drugs Don't Work*. London: Penguin Books.

Doige, Norman. 2007. *The Brain That Changes Itself: Stories of Personal Triumph from the Frontiers of Brain Science*. New York: Penguin Books.

Easterly, William. 2007. *The White Man's Burden: Why the West's Efforts to Aid the Rest Have Done So Much Ill and So Little Good*. New York: Penguin Books.

Fadiman, Anne. 2012. *The Spirit Catches You and You Fall Down: A Hmong Child, Her American Doctors, and the Collision of Two Cultures*. New York: Farrar, Straus and Giroux.

Farmer, Paul. 1999. *Infections and Inequalities: The Modern Plagues*. Berkeley: University of California Press.

Farmer, Paul. 2003. *Pathologies of Power: Health, Human Rights, and the New War on the Poor*. Berkeley: University of California Press.

Foege, William H. 2011. *House on Fire: The Fight to Eradicate Smallpox*. Berkeley: University of California Press.

Garrett, Laurie. 1994. *The Coming Plague: Newly Emerging Diseases in a World Out of Balance*. New York: Douglas & McIntyre.

Garrett, Laurie. 2001. *Betrayal of Trust: The Collapse of Global Public Health*. New York: Hyperion.

Gaskin, Ina May, and Ani DiFranco. 2011. *Birth Matters: A Midwife's Manifesta*. New York: Seven Stories Press.

Gigerenzer, Gerd, and J. A. Muir Gray, eds. 2011. *Better Doctors, Better Patients, Better Decisions: Envisioning Health Care 2020*. Cambridge, MA: MIT Press.

Gladwell, Malcolm. 2002. *The Tipping Point: How Little Things Can Make a Big Difference*. Boston: Back Bay Books.

Gleick, James. 2012. *The Information: A History, a Theory, a Flood*. New York: Vintage Books.

Glennerster, Rachel, and Kudzai Takavarasha. 2013. *Running Randomized Evaluations: A Practical Guide*. Princeton, NJ: Princeton University Press.

Gostin, Lawrence O. 2014. *Global Health Law*. Boston: Harvard University Press.

Govindarajan, Vijay, and Chris Trimble. 2012. *Reverse Innovation: Create Far From Home, Win Everywhere*. Boston: Harvard Business Review Press.

Kennedy, David. 2004. *The Dark Sides of Virtue: Reassessing International Humanitarianism*. Princeton, NJ: Princeton University Press.

Kenny, Charles. 2011. *Getting Better: Why Global Development is Succeeding—and How We Can Improve the World Even More*. New York: Basic Books.

Kidder, Tracy. 2003. *Mountains Beyond Mountains: The Quest of Dr. Paul Farmer, a Man Who would Cure the World*. New York: Random House.

Koskenniemi, Martti. 2011. *The Politics of International Law*. Portland, OR: Hart Publishing.

Kourilsky, Philippe. 2009. *Le temps de l'altruisme*. Paris: Odile Jacob.

Kuper, Andrew, ed. 2005. *Global Responsibilities: Who Must Deliver on Human Rights?* New York: Routledge.

Levine, Ruth. 2004. *Millions Saved: Proven Successes in Global Health*. Washington, DC: Center for Global Development.

Lewis, Stephen. 2005. *Race Against Time: Searching for Hope in AIDS-Ravaged Africa*. Berkeley: House of Anansi Press.

Lynch, David. 2008. *Catching the Big Fish: Meditation, Consciousness, and Creativity*. New York: Tarcher.

McNeill, William. 2010. *Plagues and Peoples*. New York: Anchor.

Moyo, Dambisa. 2009. *Dead Aid: Why Aid Is Not Working and How There Is a Better Way for Africa*. New York: Farrar, Straus and Giroux.

Neustadt, Richard E., and Harvey V. Fineberg. 1983. *The Epidemic That Never Was: Policy-Making and the Swine Flu Scare*. New York: Vintage Books.

Nolen, Stephanie. 2007. *28: Stories of AIDS in Africa*. New York: Walker & Company.

Nutt, Samantha. 2011. *Damned Nations: Greed, Guns, Armies, and Aid*. Toronto: Signal Books.

Offit, Paul A. 2007. *Vaccinated: One Man's Quest to Defeat the World's Deadliest Diseases*. Washington, DC: Smithsonian Institution Scholarly Press.

Orbinski, James. 2008. *An Imperfect Offering: Humanitarian Action in the Twenty-First Century*. Toronto: Doubleday Canada.

Piketty, Thomas. 2014. *Capital in the Twenty-First Century*. Boston: Belknap Press.

Piot, Peter. 2013. *No Time to Lose: A Life in Pursuit of Deadly Viruses*. New York: W. W. Norton.

Pogge, Thomas W. 2002. *World Poverty and Human Rights*. Cambridge, UK: Polity.

Pogge, Thomas, Matthew Rimmer, and Kim Rubenstein, eds. 2010. *Incentives for Global Public Health: Patent Law and Access to Essential Medicines*. Cambridge, UK: Cambridge University Press.

Porter, Michael E., and Elizabeth Olmsted Teisberg. 2006. *Redefining Health Care: Creating Value-Based Competition on Results*. Boston: Harvard Business Review Press.

Preston, Richard. 2002. *The Demon in the Freezer: A True Story*. New York: Random House.

Rayner, Geof, and Tim Lang. 2012. *Ecological Public Health: Reshaping the Conditions for Good Health*. New York: Routledge.

Ridley, Matt. 2010. *The Rational Optimist: How Prosperity Evolves*. New York: Harper.

Roberts, Marc, William Hsiao, Peter Berman, and Michael Reich. 2008. *Getting Health Reform Right: A Guide to Improving Performance and Equity*. New York: Oxford University Press.

Rodrik, Dani. 2010. *The Globalization Paradox: Democracy and the Future of the World Economy*. London: W. W. Norton.

Sachs, Jeffrey D. 2005. *The End of Poverty*. New York: Penguin Press.

Sell, Susan K. 2003. *Private Power, Public Law: The Globalization of Intellectual Property Rights*. Cambridge, UK: Cambridge University Press.

Shilts, Randy. 1987. *And the Band Played On: Politics, People, and the AIDS Epidemic*. New York: St. Martin's Press.

Shirley, Mary M. 2008. *Institutions and Development*. Northampton, MA: Edward Elgar Publishing.

Sims, Peter. 2011. *Little Bets: How Breakthrough Ideas Emerge from Small Discoveries*. New York: Free Press.

Spielman, Andrew, and Michael D'Antonio. 2001. *Mosquito: A Natural History of Our Most Persistent and Deadly Foe*. New York: Hyperion.

Stuckler, David, and Sanjay Basu. 2013. *The Body Economic: Why Austerity Kills*. New York: Basic Books.

Swaan, Abram de. 1999. *In Care of the State: Health Care, Education and Welfare in Europe and the USA in the Modern Era*. New York: Oxford University Press.

Tan, Chade-Meng. 2012. *Search Inside Yourself: Google's Guide to Enhancing Productivity, Creativity, and Happiness*. New York: HarperOne.

Topol, Eric. 2012. *The Creative Destruction of Medicine: How the Digital Revolution Will Create Better Health Care*. New York: Basic Books.

Tzu, Sun. 1971. *The Art of War*. Translated by Samuel B. Griffith. New York: Oxford University Press.

Walter, Chip. 2013. *Last Ape Standing: The Seven-Million-Year Story of How and Why We Survived*. London: Walker Books.

Williams, Mark, and Danny Penman. 2011. *Mindfulness: An Eight-Week Plan for Finding Peace in a Frantic World*. Emmaus, PA: Rodale Books.

INDEX